Praise for *The A-List Diet* and Dr. Pescatore

"Fred Pescatore demonstrates once again why he is one of the most innovative thinkers in the low-carb movement. This exciting and innovative new book goes way beyond the standard low-carb prescription of meat and vegetables and shows you how to make a few simple tweaks that are virtually guaranteed to get you results."

—JONNY BOWDEN, PHD, CNS, bestselling author of
The Great Cholesterol Myth, *Living Low Carb*, and *Smart Fat*

"Throughout our 25-year association, Dr. Pescatore has been the most trusted voice when it comes to my health and wellness. He has continually offered alternative and successful approaches to problems that baffled others. He is smart, sensitive, always at the forefront of what is new—and has never given up on his battle to end obesity in America. Simply put, he's a genius when it comes to diet and nutrition."

—HEIDI CLEMENTS, executive producer of *Baby Daddy*,
former executive producer of *Entertainment Tonight*,
and author of *Welcome to Heidi*

"Dr. Fred is a breed apart. He does not simply rehash what is already known in the diet world but is innovative and creative to uncover new solutions—that work. *The A-List Diet* is THE new diet book of the decade."

—ANN LOUISE GITTLEMAN, PHD, CNS, author of 30 books
on detox, health, and healing

Other Books by Fred Pescatore, MD, MPH

Feed Your Kids Well

Thin for Good

The Allergy and Asthma Cure

The Hamptons Diet

The Hamptons Diet Cookbook

Boost Your Health with Bacteria

THE
A-LIST
DIET

Lose up to *15 Pounds*
and Look and Feel Younger
in *Just 2 Weeks*

Fred Pescatore, MD, MPH

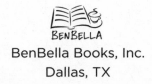

BenBella Books, Inc.
Dallas, TX

BenBella

BenBella Books, Inc.
10440 North Central Expressway, Suite 800 | Dallas, Texas 75231
www.benbellabooks.com
Send feedback to feedback@benbellabooks.com

Printed in the United States of America
10 9 8 7 6 5 4 3

Library of Congress Cataloging-in-Publication Data
Names: Pescatore, Fred, 1961- author.
Title: The a-list diet : lose up to 15 pounds and look and feel younger in
    just 2 weeks / Fred Pescatore, MD, MPH.
Description: Dallas, TX : BenBella Books, Inc. 2017. | Includes
    bibliographical references and index.
Identifiers: LCCN 2016048812 (print) | LCCN 2016049676 (ebook) | ISBN
    9781944648138 (hardback) | ISBN 9781944648145 (electronic)
Subjects: LCSH: Weight loss. | Diet. | Nutrition. | BISAC: HEALTH & FITNESS /
    Weight Loss. | HEALTH & FITNESS / Diets. | HEALTH & FITNESS /
Nutrition.
Classification: LCC RM222.2 .P43578 2017 (print) | LCC RM222.2 (ebook) |
DDC
    613.2/5--dc23
LC record available at https://lccn.loc.gov/2016048812

Editing by Vy Tran   Text design and composition by
Copyediting by Karen Wise   Silver Feather Design
Proofreading by Rachel Phares and   Front cover design by Ty Nowicki
    Cape Cod Compositors   Full cover design by Sarah Dombrowsky
Indexing by Jigsaw Information   Printed by Lake Book Manufacturing

Distributed by Perseus Distribution
www.perseusdistribution.com

To place orders through Perseus Distribution:
Tel: (800) 343-4499 | Fax: (800) 351-5073 | E-mail: orderentry@perseusbooks.com

Special discounts for bulk sales (minimum of 25 copies) are available.
Please contact Aida Herrera at aida@benbellabooks.com.

I must dedicate this book to all my patients—past, present, and future. Without each of you, I would never have made it this far. Without each of you, the world wouldn't be this savvy about health, nutrition, lifestyle, and government interference in our well-being. I have been on this journey for a long time now, and if all my patients, my readers, and my followers weren't out there supporting this movement, there would be no health food stores or organic foods in every store and on almost every menu. The giant leap of knowledge into health and nutrition was paved on your backs, on your desire to have the truth available to you no matter the cost, on your willingness to believe that perhaps the establishment doesn't know everything. I also dedicate this book to all the nutritional medical pioneers who have come before me and on whose shoulders I stand. I am happy to carry the torch for as long as someone will listen.

Together, and with all of the support from people who read and buy books of this type, we may just be starting to win the fight against the food industrial complex, giant agribusiness, Big Pharma, and their collusion with the United States government in doing their best to make us unhealthy.

Contents

PHASE THREE
Maintenance (for a Lifetime)   145

Author's Note

The information in this book reflects the author's own experience and is not intended to replace the advice of your personal physician. It is not the intent of the author to diagnose illness or prescribe treatment. The intent is only to help you lose weight and become healthier, using methods that have worked for the author's patients. Only your personal physician can determine whether this program is suitable for you, depending on your medical history. Your physician should be aware of all your medical conditions and any medications or nutritional supplements you may be taking. If you are on diuretics, diabetes medications, anti-hypertensives, or any other medication, you should proceed only under a doctor's supervision. In addition to having regular checkups and supervision, you should discuss any questions or symptoms that may arise with your personal physician.

In the event that you use the information in this book without your doctor's approval, you are prescribing for yourself and the author assumes no responsibility. As with any plan, the weight loss phases of this nutritional program should not be used by patients on dialysis or by pregnant or nursing women.

Since this diet is based on the powers of amino acids, if you have maple sugar urine disease, you absolutely cannot follow the recommendations in this book because you do not have the ability to metabolize branched-chain amino acids.

Acknowledgments

Writing a book, having a practice, and just having a life doesn't happen without the help of many people. It is with great honor that I get to mention the people who helped make *The A-List Diet* happen.

First, I would never have been an author without the help of Tom Miller, my agent. He has been encouraging me to write since my first book, *Feed Your Kids Well*. He believed in that book and every other one since. He is a great editor and now an even better agent.

I have to thank my staff at the office. Without them, I could never take the time off to write new books. They make the office hum. Carmelo Prestano, Sigalit Nisanov, Deborah Burkes, and Shantriya James—thank you for all that you do.

I also have to thank the entire staff who runs my newsletter. They keep me current, up-to-date on all the latest scientific information and help me boil it down to make it useful for everyone. They turn my ideas into actionable advice anyone can learn. The opportunities they have given me to spread the latest breakthroughs in natural health to readers like you is nothing short of incredible. Thanks to Karen Reddel, Amanda Angelini, and everyone else too numerous to mention in Batimore and beyond. It truly does take a village.

And of course, I must thank everyone at BenBella Books for giving me the opportunity to publish this book. Glenn, Monica, Vy, Heather, and the entire team have been nothing short of amazing—this has been the easiest book-writing process I have ever gone through.

Lastly, I must thank my dog Remington—who gives me solace and companionship and cheers me up when the going gets rough. Beagles rule!

Preface

Let me share how the A-List Diet was born. Toward the end of my residency training in New York City, I was completely disillusioned with medicine. I hadn't known quite what to expect during my residency, but I did know that I wanted to help people who wanted to get well. The health care system in the United States is set up to take care of those who are sick, but it does very little to teach people how to stay healthy once they get that fix. We have a really good hospital system for taking care of the catastrophic but nothing in place for those who need information to help them not get sick in the first place.

I don't know if you've ever had that feeling where you know something is off but you can't place your finger on it—that was what I felt during my residency training. It wasn't that I was tired or burned out. I simply hated what I was doing. Becoming a doctor had always been my passion, but I sure wasn't feeling any of it during those four years.

So, I decided that if I couldn't practice medicine the way I wanted to, which was to provide people with incentives and tools not to get sick, I would at least do it with my best friend from medical school in a warmer climate—on the sunny West Coast. While I waited in New York for my California medical license to be approved, I was approached to do new patient evaluations for a local doctor. His name was Dr. Robert C. Atkins. At the time, I had no idea who he was or what he had accomplished. But Dr. Atkins offered me a job and I took it—and it changed my life forever.

For the first time, I was seeing patients who actually took control of their health. They were not about to sit idly by, pop some prescription drugs, and think that was all there is to health. They didn't want to be sick—they wanted to be well. And they would do whatever it took to get that way. This involved some really radical work and thinking on their part. They had to practically forage for healthy foods. They had to learn to cook for themselves if they wanted to eat healthy. They had to learn about unfamiliar vegetables. They were encouraged to exercise, and they wouldn't take "I'm sick" for an excuse. These patients knew they could get well—they just had to find out how.

In the early 1990s, we were in the dark ages of nutritional recommendations—the low-fat era—but at the Atkins Center, my patients were focusing on fats and proteins and low-carbohydrate eating. They were going against the prevailing dogma, including eating eggs when the medical establishment claimed that cholesterol would kill you. They were eating meat and drinking martinis and getting healthier. My patients were eschewing bread and pasta when they were told by the media that they would die if they didn't eat them. They were also taking vitamins, back when supplements were still considered fringe and there was no Vitamin Shoppe on the corner. Farmers' markets weren't staples in every neighborhood, and Whole Foods Market was not a household name. If they wanted to live in a truly healthy way, they had to work at it. Keep in mind, there was also no internet with every conceivable food source and recipe at their disposal. They couldn't simply mail-order healthy foods. It was practically a full-time job to follow our advice and recommendations and, boy, were they glad that they did. These were brave souls willing to do things differently from their families, friends, and neighbors, because they knew it was healthier for them, and they wanted not only to be healthy but to stay that way.

My experience at the Atkins Center completely transformed my career. I went from a culture of illness to a culture of wellness simply by walking through that door.

I discovered that eating fat doesn't make you fat. I watched patients' cholesterol levels going down, I noticed people getting off medications rather than adding new ones, and I saw the number of people who came into our practice with diabetes leave without it. The lessons I learned from the patients in those early years have stuck with me for a lifetime.

Since my mind was clear about how medicine really should be practiced, I never ended up moving to California after all. I was thrilled with the results I was seeing with my patients and ended up staying with Dr. Atkins for five years and becoming the associate medical director of a practice that routinely saw more than two hundred patients per day. Because of our success with weight loss and with major medical concerns from diabetes to heart disease, it wasn't surprising that we cultivated quite the A-list of patients, including Stevie Nicks, Tony Curtis, Helen Gurley Brown, and a roster of American socialites and European royalty.

When I started my own practice five years later, many patients came with me. And since the A-listers are ordinary people who just happen to have extraordinary friends, my list of patients grew with each new referral. To this day, that is how my practice operates—all through word of mouth. Trust me, I have many more regular patients than celebrities, but having a celebrity endorsement means something in this country, and if it helps get my health message out, then I am all for it. I now have many more very famous patients—though since they are current patients, I can't name them.

The benefits of the low-carb lifestyle aren't limited to the rich and famous. You can be as slim and youthful looking as the most glamorous A-listers in the Hamptons, Manhattan, LA, London, Rio, St. Barths, Punta del Este, and Palm Beach. Science has been proving those of us in the low-carbohydrate camp right, over and over again. "What If It's All Been a Big Fat Lie?" was the 2002 *New York Times Magazine* cover story by Gary Taubes that changed dieting forever. From there, study after study continues to show that science validates low-carbohydrate approaches to successful weight loss.

Dr. Atkins was the master of low-carbohydrate dieting, and I learned all its secrets from him. The experience of having worked with such a visionary, who stayed true to his belief system even though the entire world thought he was crazy, changed my life. I feel blessed and honored that I have been able to continue his work and expand on it in the last two decades. I have been refining the high-protein, low-carbohydrate technique throughout my career. And if you've followed my books, you can certainly see how in each one, the science behind my ideas has evolved along with the latest nutritional research.

This developing research has led directly to the breakthrough weight-loss revolution I'm going to share with you in this book, *The A-List Diet*. A program that will help you live, feel, and look the way you want to.

Why Another Diet?

You probably know by now that eating protein and vegetables and avoiding white carbs—the basis for Paleo, Atkins, and other low-carb diet plans—is the gold standard for staying lean and thin. And I built a tremendously successful plan on this concept with my *New York Times* best seller *The Hamptons Diet*. But I have learned so much in the thirteen years since that book was published. Nutritional science has evolved rapidly since then, and I've been on top of all the cutting-edge research. I have worked with thousands of patients—including many celebrities—to lose weight and get healthy using the latest scientific advances.

Of course, it's no secret that my famous clients are fairly demanding—okay, *very* demanding. They want results fast. And the fact is, the initial honeymoon phase of low-carb eating goes away pretty quickly, especially if you are diet challenged (that is, if you have been on and off diets for years).

But thanks to my tireless research, I have found out how to give my demanding celebrity clientele maximum results from the high-protein lifestyle. Now I'm giving these tools to you. My A-list solution removes the common barriers to weight loss and gives you all the tools you will need for weight loss success—and optimal long-term health.

The A-List Diet goes beyond Atkins, beyond the Hamptons and South Beach, beyond Virgin, beyond Zero Belly, beyond Wheat

Belly, and beyond Paleo. Grounded in the latest cutting-edge science, this diet will have you looking good on the inside, which makes you look better on the outside—the natural way. I have been in practice for more than twenty years, and the A-List Diet gives quite simply the most amazing results that I have seen in my entire career.

The key is *PROTEIN BOOSTING*.

Customized protein boosting turbocharges your weight loss as you become leaner and fitter, and it also helps slow down the aging process. My A-list patients look great largely due to the fact that they are aging more slowly from within.

Amanda's A-List Diet Story

My patient Amanda is a Golden Globe Award winner. She needed to lose about ten pounds before the 2015 Golden Globes ceremony, which took place shortly after the end-of-the-year holidays. Amanda has been working with me for quite some time, but with all the pressure on her that year, she took partying to a new level in Punta del Este, Uruguay. Yes, she was in an exciting place, eating delicious new foods, relaxing for hours lying on the beach, and drinking exotic drinks, but adding ten pounds right before red carpet season might not have been the optimal thing to do.

Luckily, I knew how she usually ate, so all I needed to do was simply protein boost her, in addition to adjusting the proteins in her meals. Within two weeks, she had lost the ten pounds—in plenty of time for the show. She didn't even have to adjust her exercise regimen. She looked fabulous when she picked up her award, and she *felt* even better.

WHAT IS PROTEIN BOOSTING?

Protein boosting simply uses the powers of amino acids—the building blocks of all proteins—to help speed your metabolism, decrease inflammation, and get you off any plateau you may be experiencing. There are twenty-two major amino acids in the human body, hundreds of minor amino acids, and three of them are the most crucial to the weight loss process. In this book I will show you step by step how to incorporate these three vital amino acids into your diet through foods, drinks, shakes, and supplements—and by rotating the proteins in your meals and menu plans. The other amino acids are important for your health and well-being, too, but these three hold the key to your weight loss dreams.

LOSE UP TO FIVE POUNDS A WEEK UNTIL YOU REACH YOUR GOAL WEIGHT

I know you're looking for the numbers, so here they are. You can lose five pounds a week on this diet, sometimes more. I have had patients lose seven to ten pounds in one week. But keep in mind that it's easiest to lose weight at the beginning of any diet. So, after the first two weeks (the first week is Phase One, the second week and beyond is Phase Two), I would expect you to lose an average of two or three pounds per week, which is a sensible and successful way to lose weight until you reach your goal and then maintain it.

Celebrities are all about an unrealistic version of skinniness, which shouldn't be our main goal. It is, after all, their job to make the rest of us look bad while being that aspirational model that we know deep down is not possible. For someone who has worked with these people, I can tell you that you are either born genetically blessed or have to be very drastic in terms of food and exercise in order to achieve those goal—and more often than not, both. While I can help you with the dieting portion of how the A-listers stay slim, and you will even get some tips on how to enhance your genetics, the exercise and other enhancements that they do for themselves are not what you will find in this book. Be happy with the weight you lose. Even my male A-listers want to achieve their birth weight, and this is an unrealistic goal for us normal folk. So here is a little advice before we get started: If you have never been thin in your life, choose an A-lister you think looks great and is around your height and shoot for that person's target weight. Even seemingly unrealistic weight loss goals are attainable through this diet because of the metabolic advantage you gain through protein boosting. The protein boost never fails!

However, my advice to you is try to be realistic and do this diet in a healthy way. I'm not going to set your weight loss goals for you. I know you want to lose weight to look terrific, but in truth, you should get healthy and let the weight loss be a side effect—that's the doctor in me speaking. If I had to give you some guidelines, you may want to use the body mass index (BMI)—there are plenty of apps to help you figure out your ideal weight—or else you can consult your health care practitioner. I readily admit the BMI is not the perfect tool, but it can certainly give you a "sense" of where you want your weight to be to achieve optimal health. In any case, ideally you should set your own goals based on what you want to achieve, not some unrealistic vision of skinniness. Both your waistline and your health will thank you.

Let's get started!

CHAPTER ONE

Five Secrets to Weight Loss Success

T his chapter will explain the five secrets to fast—and lasting—weight loss success that every other diet is missing. The five secrets are as follows:

1. Amino acids
2. Protein boosts
3. Inflammation
4. Alkalization
5. DNA/epigenetics

As a doctor, I can't isolate the benefits of weight loss and proper weight management from the benefits you will gain in health. Heart disease, obesity, diabetes, and the other illnesses that are epidemic in our society can all be traced back to the way we eat. If we can eat our way into these diseases, we can eat our way out of them.

But first, let me answer these simple questions, which are the keys to the A-List Diet: What are amino acids? What are protein boosts? What's inflammation got to do with dieting? What is alkalization, and what can it do for you? How can your genetics help you lose weight?

WHAT ARE AMINO ACIDS?

Twenty percent of the human body is made up of protein, and amino acids are the buildings blocks of all proteins. Protein plays a crucial role in almost all biological processes, and that's what makes amino acids the very foundation of your body, necessary for building and maintaining your muscles and vital organs. I've found that adding certain amino acids to your supplement arsenal and getting them from the foods you eat is absolutely essential if you want to lose weight.

Not only are amino acids the basis of all life processes, but they are also necessary for every metabolic process, hence their crucial role in weight loss. They are responsible for the optimal transport and storage of all nutrients (water, fat, carbohydrates, proteins, minerals, and vitamins). Amino acids can also be used as a source of energy by the body, and this is why protein boosting is the key to supercharged weight loss.

AMINO ACID SCIENCE

Amino acids are classified into three groups: essential amino acids, nonessential amino acids, and conditional amino acids. The body cannot make essential amino acids, so they have to come from the food you eat. And, if you aren't rotating your proteins, are vegetarian/vegan, or are simply not eating enough protein or getting your protein from poor sources, you are likely to lack these crucial elements for a supercharged metabolism. The nine essential amino acids are histidine, isoleucine, leucine, lysine, methionine, phenylalanine, threonine, tryptophan, and valine.

On the other hand, our bodies can produce nonessential amino acids, even if we do not get them from our diet. This group includes alanine, asparagine, aspartic acid, and glutamic acid. Finally, conditional amino acids are typically not essential, and can be made in the body except in times of illness or stress. These include arginine, cysteine, glutamine, glycine, ornithine, proline, taurine, serine, and tyrosine.

A large proportion of our cells, muscles, and tissues are made up of amino acids, so they help give cells their structure. Amino acids have an influence on the function of organs, glands, tendons, and arteries. They are also essential for healing wounds and repairing tissue, especially in the muscles, bones, skin, and hair, as well as for the removal of all kinds of waste deposits produced in connection with metabolism.

Getting the amino acid balance just right is the future of low-carb, higher-protein diets.

It's not enough to just eat higher amounts of protein and lower amounts of carbohydrates. Many scientists are confirming that a supply of amino acids (from either the right foods or nutritional supplements) can have positive effects. This is the missing link in all the other higher-protein diets out there, including my previous diet book, *The Hamptons Diet.* Science is changing constantly, and I want to help you keep up with the latest findings so you can lose weight and feel healthier.

Unfortunately, countless factors are working to prevent our bodies from receiving a full and balanced supply of these all-important aminos. Among these factors are the pollution caused by burning fossil fuels, the hormones fed to cattle, the intensive use of herbicides and fertilizers in agriculture, and even habits such as smoking and drinking—all of which can prevent our bodies from fully using what we eat or extracting all the nutritional value from a particular food. Worse still is the amount of nutrition that is lost from our food through processing before we actually get to eat it. By providing the body with optimal nutrition, amino acids help replace those lost nutrients and promote weight loss, well-being, and vitality.

The proportion of the different amino acids in what we eat or supplement have to be just right, since the aminos in our bodies are partially responsible for helping us achieve a balanced metabolism.

That may be why some of the other higher-protein diets didn't work for you or didn't get you to your goal or didn't help you stay that way—they didn't focus on amino acid balancing. It's why the A-List Diet will succeed where others failed. Science is now revealing amino acid balance and gut health to be the two cornerstones of optimal health and weight management. And by following the advice laid out in this book, you can achieve both.

DIP YOUR FOOT INTO
THE AMINO ACID POOL

The amino acid pool describes the entire amount of available free amino acids in the human body. The size of the pool amounts to 120 to 130 grams in an adult male. When we consume protein, the gastrointestinal tract breaks it down into the individual amino acids and then puts them back together again as new protein in a complex biological process called protein biosynthesis. This delicate balance can be thrown off by eating the wrong proteins, the wrong combination of proteins, or damaged (that is, nonorganic) proteins. The entire amino acid pool is transformed, or "exchanged," three to four times a day. This means that the body has to be regularly supplied with more amino acids, partly through protein biosynthesis and partly through what we eat or take in via supplementation.

The amino acids in the pool need to be maintained in the correct combination. If one or more amino acids are not available in sufficient quantities, the production of protein is weakened and metabolic function may be limited. This is precisely where those other higher-protein diets fail to deliver. They just advise you to eat more protein, when the answer is to eat the right protein for your metabolic needs (or, as I describe it in the next chapter, your "dieting type").

And if the amino acid pool isn't maintained properly, guess what happens? Weight problems, hair loss, skin concerns, sleep disorders, mood swings, and/or erectile disorders. Not to mention arthritis, diabetes, cardiovascular imbalance (high cholesterol levels, high blood pressure), or even menopausal complaints. We are mostly going to focus on the weight problems in this book, but as I often tell my patients, weight loss is simply a side effect of good health.

I think this intrinsic need for proper protein balance is the main reason why diets higher in protein have been adopted by many people around the world. And when you think about it, in just a few years, higher-protein diets have accomplished what the government, albeit in a feeble effort, has failed to do in decades, and that is to convince us that grains, especially refined grains, are bad for us. Millions of people now shun unhealthy foods such as white bread, mega-muffins, giant bagels, pizza crusts, sweets, white rice, and white pasta.

In addition to the guidelines in this book, there is an enormous amount of literature out there, backed by real science, that will help you learn what you should and shouldn't be eating. I've found with my patients that when they know why they're doing what they're doing, it helps them stay on track.

MY FAVORITE AMINOS:
THE PROTEIN BOOSTERS

I have been successfully using the tenets of what I wrote about in *The Hamptons Diet* for about fifteen years. Since the diet was so successful, there was no reason to tamper with it until now. I have been in the nutrition business for more than twenty years, and the one thing I did learn in that time is that science doesn't sit still. I write a free e-newsletter called the Reality Health Check, which I encourage you to sign up for to get the latest, breaking health news (see the Resources section to find out how). I bring this up because it was while researching the material for one of these e-letters that I discovered the impact of branched-chain amino acids (BCAAs) in boosting metabolism. In fact, the research on BCAAs is so compelling that I've taken to thinking of them as the missing link between health and weight loss.

The BCAAs are leucine, isoleucine, and valine. These three little substances are going to help you lose weight like you have never done before. In one study, BCAAs were administered to patients on a high-fat, high-protein diet. In just six weeks, those taking the BCAAs had 7 percent less body weight and 49 percent less white adipose tissue. Not only that, their livers held less triglycerides (what I like to call "stowaway sugar"). Lower triglyceride levels play an important role in keeping your heart healthy and preventing heart attacks and strokes—even more so than your cholesterol level. Another study found lowered triglycerides in patients given BCAAs, as well as a 47 percent reduction in the degree of hyperinsulinism, an important biomarker for metabolic disrepair.

BCAAs have also been shown to increase "fat-free mass" or, in other words, to promote a leaner you after just thirty days. Most diets lead you toward calorie restriction (especially the big diets with a lot of money behind them), but in most circles, it has not been proven that all calories are not the same. The effects of a calorie on your metabolism depend on its micronutrient structure—for example, a calorie from sugar does not give your body the same benefit as a calorie from wild salmon. The A-List Diet does not restrict calories but instead focuses on nutrient-dense foods and, in turn, opens up a world of food possibilities that you never knew could exist in a diet program.

Furthermore, when you restrict calories, you tend to lose lean muscle. One of the BCAAs, leucine, has been shown to initiate protein synthesis in muscles and to help regulate blood sugar levels by promoting muscle uptake of floating blood sugar. It is able to improve insulin sensitivity primarily by decreasing body fat. By working in this way, leucine may help decrease your chances of getting diabetes. And this wonder-amino helps you retain that lean muscle mass.

Elite wrestlers, for instance, supplement their diets with BCAAs, which leads to significant losses of abdominal visceral fat. That's right—taking BCAAs can get rid of that stubborn belly fat. That's why my patients love the A-List Diet. And you will, too.

There are dozens more studies showing just how many things BCAAs can do for us. It is really when I started to see all this literature that I knew I could help my patients overcome their biggest weight loss and health challenges simply by correcting one thing— their amino acid balance. It changed my practice and it will change your life.

OTHER AMINO ACID WEIGHT LOSS PLAYERS

Whether we gradually put on weight or stay slim depends on our hormones. I've discovered, at least in my practice, that the key to weight loss is the systematic supplementation of certain amino acids that allow us to stimulate the body to produce enough fat-burning hormones in a natural manner.

One important fat-burning hormone that you don't hear too much about is the growth hormone somatotropin. Unless you live in the world of body builders, or have done significant research in the anti-aging literature, you probably haven't heard of it. But it's critical in helping you lose weight.

Somatotropin is produced while we sleep—which is why sleeping disorders often lead to weight gain or obesity. This hormone stimulates protein synthesis and boosts fat oxidation. Sadly, overweight patients have lower somatotropin concentrations to begin with. I have many patients who inject growth hormone as part of their healthy lifestyle regimen, but that is very expensive and does have potential side effects, such as muscle and joint pain and maybe even cancer. Besides, many people don't like needles, and the effectiveness is not any better than the protein boosts I've included in the A-List Diet, which quite literally mimic the effects of the injections without the expense and pain.

The amino acids glutamine, arginine, and methionine (along with vitamins B_6 and B_{12} and zinc) can also help synthesize growth hormone in your body. In fact, they're known as growth hormone secretagogues. They are effective when taken religiously, in high dosages at bedtime. However, they aren't as effective as the protein boosts.

Glutamine and Fat Storage

Glutamine can be converted to glucose in the kidneys without affecting glucagon and insulin, the two hormones responsible for blood sugar regulation. Therefore, it stops insulin from storing fat and helps regulate weight. Glutamine can also reduce cravings for sugar and alcohol. Combining it with vitamin B is especially helpful since almost all the B vitamins stimulate the body's ability to break down fat (B_2, B_3, B_5, B_7, and B_{12} appear to be particularly effective). Zinc is also necessary in this process since it supports the body in processing fats and carbohydrates. In fact, the amino acids can do their job only with a sufficient supply of zinc.

Glutamine has been shown to improve insulin resistance while improving adipose mass, a downward trend in blood pressure, a decrease in fasting blood sugar, a decrease in HgbA1c levels (a measure of how well your blood sugar is controlled over a six-week period), a leaner body composition, and weight loss.

Carnitine: Another Unsung Hero

Carnitine is synthesized in the liver (and its precursor in the kidneys) from the amino acids lysine and methionine. It acts on the mitochondria, which are the energy-producing parts of each cell. The more carnitine that is around, the more quickly fatty acids get burned instead of stored. Carnitine basically stokes the furnace. It is abundant in red meat and dairy products and helps your body convert fat into energy. The proper synthesis of carnitine involves vitamins B_6 and B_{12}, niacin, and folic acid. If there is a deficiency in any of these vitamins, you won't be able to make enough carnitine to keep your body a lean machine.

Study after study shows the effect of carnitine on fat oxidation, protein usage, body composition, weight management, fatigue, hunger, and the metabolic syndrome. But there are also studies that show us that carnitine may help combat angina, heart attack, heart failure, peripheral vascular disease (and intermittent claudication, in particular), diabetic neuropathy, Alzheimer's disease, depression, memory loss, male infertility, and erectile dysfunction.

The amino acids are going to be our friends in the pursuit of weight loss and health, partially by providing the building blocks for keeping our bodies doing what they need to do internally and partially by their very nature as metabolic repair heroes.

Now, let's discuss the next hidden factor that may be keeping you from reaching your weight loss goals.

INFLAMMATION AND ITS EFFECT ON WEIGHT LOSS

Any way you look at it, there is but one bottom line: Inflammation is the cause of most, if not all, illnesses. Chronic inflammation will also prevent you from losing weight; that's why I spend so much time discussing it.

So where does all this inflammation come from? It basically comes from living in the toxic environment we've set up for ourselves. We live in a world of endocrine disruptors, antibiotic residue in the foods we eat, and polluted and nutrient-depleted soil, not to mention the usual suspects such as air and water pollution. And let's not forget about stress. While you may say you don't feel stressed, trust me, your body does. And your body does the best it can to spare you the ravages of this constant stress until it can't anymore. And weight gain or the inability to manage your weight is one of the first signs.

Our national dependency on sugar is a huge contributor to chronic inflammation. The A-List Diet removes this very toxic food substance from your diet. So if you are squeamish about the thought of giving up your "favorite" foods, then stop reading right now. But, while giving up sugar may seem like an insurmountable task, consider this: It takes only three days.

Once you can get past the seventy-two-hour mark, your physiological craving for sugar goes away and you are left with just the psychological craving. I am not going to say that the psychological craving can't be difficult to overcome, but getting rid of the physiological craving makes dealing with your psyche a lot easier. And take it from me—a former overweight person whose favorite food was (and still is) ice cream—there isn't a day that goes by that I don't still think of eating it. But it's only on very rare occasions that I ever actually do. I mention this to show you that it's okay to think about unhealthy foods as long as you're not frequently acting on those thoughts.

THE DIFFERENCE BETWEEN "GOOD" AND "BAD" INFLAMMATION

In itself, inflammation is a good thing. It's how your body protects and heals itself. Without it, wounds and infections would never get better. Any time you injure yourself or are exposed to some sort of infection, your immune system responds by sending out substances called "inflammatory mediators." Histamine, prostaglandins, and cytokines are probably the most well-known.

Inflammatory mediators increase blood flow. They also allow more white blood cells to get through your blood vessel walls to the site of the infection or injury. All of this is necessary to heal you. But in the process, it can also cause redness, fever, swelling, and—yes—pain. This sort of response is known as acute inflammation. And it generally goes away on its own within a few days (at the most).

On the flip side, when inflammation is too active or doesn't go away, it can make us sick. We know that major chronic illnesses, such as heart disease and type 2 diabetes, are linked to weight gain, and in turn to inflammation.

Chronic inflammation generally makes your life miserable. This is the inflammation that causes arthritis pain, fibromyalgia, allergies, back pain, and so on. And if you don't rein it in, it can lead to more serious conditions such as heart disease, cancer, and Alzheimer's disease, to name but a few.

But as complicated as the inflammatory process is, keeping it under control is actually quite simple. Like most health problems, the best place to start battling inflammation is with food. Eating an unhealthy diet, not exercising enough, and consuming too much sugar can contribute to chronic inflammation. These poor habits turn the immune system "on" and help it stay activated for a long period of time, causing problems rather than eliminating them.

In fact, I'd go so far as to say inflammation is a full-on crisis. And decreasing it should be priority number one. The A-List Diet is, at its core, an anti-inflammatory diet. Once you are able to conquer inflammation, the rest of your health will fall into place.

CHRONIC INFLAMMATION AND WEIGHT GAIN

The main reason we suffer from chronic inflammation comes down to the dreadful diet that's become the "standard" in this country. The Standard American Diet (SAD) relies heavily on packaged, processed foods that contain many inflammatory substances. And here's the rub: Once you become obese or overweight, that compounds the inflammation problem even more. Body fat, especially belly fat, triggers a low-grade ongoing inflammatory process throughout the body. To prove this point, a study from the UK published in 2008 shows that weight increases were associated with more inflammation, and the relationship was linear. This means that as a person's weight increased, so did the level of C-reactive protein (CRP) in their blood.

CRP is a blood marker for inflammation that you can ask your doctor to measure for you. I measure it for all my patients and have found it very useful in managing their weight loss and other related health conditions. You can watch this marker go down as you lose weight and become healthier and less inflamed.

Take "Out" the "In"flammation

Here are six tips for lowering inflammation (and note that the A-List Diet program does all this for you):

1. **Eat antioxidants and polyphenols:** Eating antioxidant- and polyphenol-rich foods can cut down on inflammation by reducing "free-radical damage." Free radicals are generated by the body when it's in a state of stress. If the immune system becomes overwhelmed by free radicals, cells are harmed and inflammation gets worse. To get antioxidants and polyphenols, eat a rainbow of fruits and veggies, like broccoli, kale, collards, and berries.

2. **Consume essential fats:** Getting a good ratio of omega-6 and omega-3 fatty acids in your diet is important for reducing inflammation. Most of us consume too much omega-6 and not enough omega-3, so the key to balancing things is to increase your omega-3 intake. Omega-6-heavy foods like refined vegetable oils (used in many snack foods, crackers, and cookies) tend to stir up inflammation, while foods high in omega-3s, like salmon, flaxseed, chia seeds, avocado, and walnuts, dampen it.

3. **Add spices:** Turmeric, garlic, cinnamon, cayenne pepper, and ginger have all been shown in studies to have anti-inflammatory properties. You can't overdo these, so sprinkle them liberally on your food.

4. **Exercise:** Moving around releases a burst of anti-inflammatory proteins. However, moderate exercise is key. An example of moderate exercise is forty to sixty minutes of cardio, such as walking or jogging, about three times a week. The science of exercise is probably moving more quickly than the science of nutrition, and at the moment, most studies are pointing to exercise in moderation as the right amount to strive for, in terms of health-related benefits.

5. **De-stress:** Cortisol regulates the immune response. Reducing stress helps keep hormones like cortisol under control and that, in turn, helps lower inflammation.

6. **Sleep:** There is a complex yet harmonious dance occurring in your body during restful sleep; this strengthens your immune system.

The A-List Diet will help you lower your chronic level of inflammation. My patients feel better within a few days of starting the program. Their energy level improves, sleep gets better, and an overall sense of well-being increases—all things you can expect to feel from the moment you start the program. It's as simple as changing what you eat and getting in those protein boosts.

THE ALKALIZATION SECRET

Alkalization is an important part of the A-List Diet strategy. The pH scale ranges from 0 (acid) to 14 (alkaline), with 7 being perfectly neutral. While various parts of your body maintain different pH levels, your blood's natural pH is always slightly alkaline, around 7.36.

Good health depends on maintaining this pH balance. It keeps your body in its ideal state and maximizes the functioning of all your systems. But the typical American diet does nothing to support that goal. In fact, it tips the scales toward acidity. And that, in turn, promotes excess inflammation, weight gain, and disease states.

While the A-List Diet tends to focus on amino acids, and amino acids tend toward the acidic range, I emphasize foods and provide protein boosts and shakes that keep your pH balanced and in check. Other low-carb, high-protein diets on the bestseller lists fail to do that and keep you in a constant state of acidity.

What determines whether a food is considered alkaline or acidic depends on the residue—known as "ash"—that food leaves behind after it is metabolized. If it leaves an acidic ash it is an acidic food, and vice versa. So if you eat foods that create acidic ash, it makes your body acidic. If you eat foods that turn into alkaline ash, it makes your body alkaline. Neutral ash has no effect. Simple.

Acidic ash is produced by meat, poultry, cheese, fish, eggs, and grains. Alkaline ash is produced by fruits and vegetables, except cranberries, prunes, and plums. Foods such as citrus fruits that are generally considered acidic are actually alkaline since that is the residue left behind after those are metabolized.

Here's what you should know about alkaline foods:

1. They reduce inflammation.
2. They promote clearer thinking (less "brain fog").
3. They promote effective circulation of blood and lymph.
4. They help reduce allergies.

5. They help maintain an even distribution of energy throughout the body.
6. They support overall calmness.

Here's what you should know about acidic foods:

1. They promote inflammation.
2. They cause muscle aches, generalized pains, and joint pains.
3. They cause brain and body fatigue.
4. They promote foggy brain.
5. They cause indigestion and poor elimination.
6. They prevent effective blood and lymph circulation.
7. They cause wounds to heal more slowly.

You don't need to remember or test your pH numbers as part of the A-List Diet protocols. By simply taking stock of your own symptoms you can usually tell. The bottom line: If you just don't feel well, your body's probably generating more acid than it should be.

As we get further into the nitty-gritty of the diet itself, I will have lists that outline which foods are more alkaline and which are more acidic. Maintaining your pH balance, which my A-List Diet does so effectively, keeps your body in its ideal metabolic state and maximizes the functioning of all your systems. You'll be as fit and thin as the A-list celebrities and look and feel years younger than you ever thought possible.

TAP INTO YOUR DNA: THE GENETIC LINK TO WEIGHT LOSS

Your genetics can help you lose weight or gain it. The A-List Diet is here to turn the weight loss genes on and the weight gain genes off. Your DNA has the potential to dictate an optimal diet for you as well as optimal exercise to maximize your body's potential.

Nick's A-List Story

Nick, a good-looking Italian-American guy from Queens, came to see me because he worked out, thought he was eating right (he was a big fan of my previous book, *The Hamptons Diet*), *but* he still had a gut. He carried about twenty-five pounds around the middle, and there was certainly room for toning. He said to me, "Doc, I don't know why I'm here. I read your newsletter and I think I know what you're going to tell me, but I need some extra help." Well, six weeks later and thirty pounds lighter, he was very glad he came to see me in person.

After examining his blood work and what he ate, it was clear to me why the typical meat, fish, and vegetable diet wasn't working for him. He was eating too much of the wrong proteins, creating inflammation, causing insulin resistance, and making his body too acidic for weight loss.

That's where most people go wrong when they embark on high-protein diets—they eat any protein they want and don't realize the importance of getting the balance right.

So I moved Nick from chicken eggs to quail eggs, and I substituted more alkaline vegetables, such as collard greens instead of spinach and endive instead of zucchini. Most importantly, I added amino acids to his program in the form of protein boosts. He consumed the protein boosts twice per day as I recommended, and it was this change that jump-started his metabolism and leaned him out.

Nick's story ends really well: He is about to get married to a very famous singer he met at my office.

This aspect of nutritional science is called nutrigenetics (which, along with epigenetics and nutrigenomics, are all terms used interchangeably at this point), and it is the cutting-edge science of nutrition, weight, and fitness. Genetics dictates our hair and eye color, and it also dictates how we metabolize nutrients, the way our body handles toxins, and how poorly or well we interact with what the environment throws our way.

Although we are not slaves to our genetic makeup, our genes interact with the environment, and this interaction may cause our genes to express themselves differently. Epigenetics are changes on the genome that are copied from one cell generation to the next, which may alter gene expression, but which do not involve changes in the primary DNA sequence.

Wouldn't it be nice to be able to blame your genetics for why you are fat? While there is more and more evidence that points to that conclusion, it is not a fait accompli that you will be overweight if you come from an obese family. I come from a family of obese and diabetic individuals. And I was obese. I changed that by changing the way I eat forever. But I can gain weight more quickly than most and have to watch what I eat all the time. There is no way around that yet. While we are starting to uncover the role of epigenetics, we are still a long way off from having that magic bullet to help you lose weight rapidly, easily, and forever. Until then, we have the A-List Diet program.

In fact, the foods that I recommend were specifically chosen for their ability to combat the part of your genetics that are associated with weight gain and metabolic syndromes. The A-List Diet is based in part on the study of how the nutrients (or lack thereof) in the food you eat influence the expression of your genes.

The major part of epigenetics that is associated with nutrition and dieting is telomere length. Telomeres are the ends of the strands of our DNA. Until very recently, they were thought to have no use. Now we know they act as a barrier to cellular degradation. Think of telomeres as the plastic tips of your shoelaces. Once those tips fall off, the shoelace begins to unravel and you can't tie your shoe. In the case of DNA, we get only a finite number of times the cell can replicate, and if those telomere ends aren't intact, the cells will die more quickly, leading to poor health and nutrition.

So, let's say you've turned on those fat genes—now what happens? The fat cells will release adipokines, which leads to inflammation, which turns off your satiety hormones. Then you start to crave carbohydrates, which feeds the fat cells and you accumulate more visceral fat. Visceral fat accumulates around your organs and is the deadliest type of fat because it grows by stealing the fuel supply of your muscles.

Dietary exposures can have consequences for health years or decades later, and this raises questions about the mechanisms through which such exposures are "remembered" and how they result in altered disease risk. There is growing evidence that numerous dietary factors can modify epigenetic traits. Our genetic variations have been demonstrated in recent research to affect our uptake, transport, metabolism, and elimination of food components. Our genes also determine our individual daily requirements for some essential nutrients—the amino acids found in the protein boosts, for example.

Most of us don't know our genetic make-up. There are genetic tests available, but I don't actually use them in my practice. I feel that if you're eating a healthy diet, exercising, and getting enough sleep, there's really no need to know about your genetics and stress about them. I do understand that knowing could be a motivating factor for some, but I am a strong advocate of self-motivation in the case of healthier living. Being healthier, stronger, and living longer should motivate you enough.

Besides, eating more fruits and vegetables just makes sense from a health standpoint, regardless of whether you have a genetic tendency toward weight gain. They've all got something to offer: asparagus, arugula, artichoke hearts, berries of all sorts, endive, escarole, melons, shallots, spinach, sprouts, yard-long beans, and zucchini—and everything in between. Experiment with fruits and vegetables you've never tried before, and eat even more of your old favorites. Your genes and your waistline will thank you for it.

The way you eat is the true cornerstone of your health. I can recommend all the drugs and supplements in the world, but if your diet isn't up to snuff in a consistent way, you can't expect to see real results. Every dieter who has been successful knows it's about making changes to your lifestyle for the long haul.

The true beginning of diet is nutrition and the micro- and macro-nutrients of the foods that you eat. That's why an anti-inflammatory, alkalizing diet serves as the foundation of my weight loss strategies. There is no other diet out there that takes all this into account. We are learning how to make changes to our bodies down to the cellular level, and the A-List Diet will be the first to deal with this without complicated menus and DNA testing. The A-List Diet also brings you the breakthrough amino acid boosts that have been revolutionary in my practice and for my patients. I can't wait to hear how it helps you, too.

CHAPTER TWO

What Type of Dieter Are You?

n all of my years of treating those who need to lose weight, I have found that there is no "one diet fits all." That's why I've identified six different types of A-list dieters:

1. A perimenopausal woman
2. A woman in her twenties or thirties
3. A menopausal or postmenopausal woman
4. A young man (in his twenties or thirties)
5. An andropausal man over forty
6. A diet-challenged woman or man (you've been going on and off diets for years)

While some of these categories may overlap, choose the one that best fits you for the stage of life you are in. While many of us consider ourselves diet challenged, many of us have never needed to lose weight before. So, simply opt for the category that best suits you at this exact moment in time—you can always change later depending on your level of success.

The actual food portion of the programs won't vary too greatly, so don't be alarmed. And I will outline that in the coming chapters. In this chapter, we'll focus on profiles of the different dieter types, as well as the protein booster shakes for each. The protein booster shakes are crucial for enabling your dieting type to function as an efficient metabolic fat-burning machine. Each shake varies according to your dieting type because we need different amino acids and other nutritional supplements depending on the interplay between our hormones, metabolism, and the macronutrients (proteins, fats, and carbs) that we need at any given time in our lives. These shakes are what will make a lower-carbohydrate diet work for you. They are the missing link to jump-charge your metabolism.

Note that all amino acids in the recipes are available at any supplement store, and the BCAA powders come in a variety of flavors to suit your taste. Most BCAA powders will come in a ratio of 2:1:1 of leucine to isoleucine to valine. You can find one with a 4:1:1 ratio, which is even better. Look for a blend where one scoop yields a minimum of 3,000 mg of leucine and then adjust your dose by adding multiple scoops according to the following recipes. Some BCAA formulas will include glutamine, which will also help to make things easier.

THE PERIMENOPAUSAL WOMAN

A perimenopausal woman is someone generally between the ages of forty-three and fifty-three. Perimenopause starts long before any missed periods. This is the time in a woman's life when her nicely balanced hormones really begin to fluctuate even if she has no menopausal symptoms.

This transitional period of time before menopause may cause serious distress. Symptoms of perimenopause can begin as early as ten to fifteen years before menses completely stop. Women in their late thirties, forties, and early fifties may transition in and out of a perimenopausal state many times before they finally enter menopause. Some of the most common symptoms are moodiness, fuzzy thinking, short-term memory issues, lack of focus, fatigue, head-aches, weight gain, menstrual irregularities of any sort, sleep issues, and many others. I treat many women in this time of their lives and it can indeed be challenging. If you happen to be in this group, don't beat yourself up about it—simply do something about it.

Stop and Pay Attention to Yourself!

American women have hormonal levels that tend towards higher estrogen (which, incidentally, is likely the reason one in eight women get breast cancer). This is due to a diet higher in simple carbs and lower in quality protein and unbalanced amino acids, not enough nutrients from the food you eat, not enough healthy fats and too many unhealthy ones, and, of course, environmental toxins and excess hormones from the foods you eat—all potential endocrine and meta-bolic disruptors.

During perimenopause, it is the fluctuation of estrogen (and its relationship to other hormones such as progesterone) that causes the difficulties. Fat is one of the places where the body stores estrogen. So, as your estrogen levels decrease, the body likes to hold on to the fat in order to have an extra supply of estrogen. Perimenopause is a double or even triple whammy on your metabolism.

That's why this is the hardest category to find yourself in. It is probably the most difficult and challenging time to lose weight in a woman's life. When I see patients in this age group, they fall into one of two subgroups. The first are those women who have been thin their entire lives, so dieting is a new concept for them. These women pose the most difficult challenge since they aren't used to dieting and have to learn a new skill.

The second subgroup are the women who have gained weight with pregnancies and just never got around to taking it all off or women who have put on about ten pounds per decade. Whatever subgroup you belong to, the A-List Diet has you covered.

Here is the protein booster shake recipe for perimenopausal women:

Protein Booster Shake
for the Perimenopausal Woman

3,000 mg L-leucine
750 mg L-valine
750 mg L-isoleucine
7,500 mg L-glutamine
2,000 mg L-carnitine
1 tablespoon macadamia nut oil
1 tablespoon freshly ground chia seeds
1 teaspoon ground turmeric
¼ cup unsweetened coconut or almond milk
6 ice cubes

Combine all the ingredients in a blender and puree until smooth.

A Note on the Ingredients

Since there are commonalities to the shakes, I would like to explain why various ingredients are there in the first place. Where there is a variation as we go through the A-List dieter types, I will explain it in the respective section. The branched-chain amino acids combination (leucine, isoleucine, and valine) is a good dose for women. The large dose of glutamine is for additional sugar craving support and to maintain and heal any potential gut issues. The carnitine is for turbo-charging your metabolism. The macadamia nut oil gives a metabolism boost. The chia seeds serve two purposes—they are an amazing source of fiber, so your detox will be effective and toxins will continue to be eliminated, and they are a good source of omega-3 fats. The turmeric is to reduce inflammation. The unsweetened coconut or almond milk makes the shake taste good while adding some vitamins and minerals.

THE WOMAN IN HER TWENTIES OR THIRTIES

For women, this is the sweet spot for weight loss. It is a relatively easy task to manage weight in this period, but still there are some obstacles. The biggest challenge for the women that I treat is the juggling of their career, home life, children, pregnancy, and breastfeeding. This diet and the recommended nutritional supplements is not intended for women who are pregnant or breastfeeding—these are just two obstacles in your attempt to stay thin and healthy.

Many women in this group are already used to exercising, so that will make weight loss easier. Truly, the main thing to be concerned about is following the program consistently. The A-List Diet should come easily to you.

However, it's not all wine and roses in this age group. You often have to face taking off the "freshman fifteen," the desire to be dangerously skinny for your wedding, and the inevitable catastrophic metabolic destruction of calorie restriction. Hormones will also try to interfere with your weight loss at this stage in your life. While they should be fairly balanced, oral contraceptives, pregnancy, and breast-feeding are all sources of potential hormonal imbalances.

My piece of advice for losing the baby weight (although I'm not an obstetrician) is that the new rule of thumb is to gain only about twenty pounds during pregnancy. This will decrease your risk for long-term weight issues but will especially decrease your likelihood of getting gestational diabetes. Should that occur, you are facing a life-long struggle with weight and insulin resistance issues.

Here is the protein booster shake recipe for women in their twenties and thirties:

Protein Booster Shake for the Woman in Her Twenties and Thirties

3,000 mg L-leucine
750 mg L-valine
750 mg L-isoleucine
4,000 mg L-glutamine
1 tablespoon macadamia nut oil
1 tablespoon freshly ground chia seeds
1 tablespoon freshly ground flaxseed
¼ cup unsweetened coconut or almond milk
6 ice cubes

Combine all the ingredients in a blender and puree until smooth.

A Note on the Ingredients

While it's easier for women in their twenties and thirties to lose weight, I still included the glutamine in this recipe since we can all use a little bit of help to curb our cravings. The only new ingredient here is flaxseed for additional fiber and its special fatty acid called GLA, which helps in hormonal regulation.

THE MENOPAUSAL OR POSTMENOPAUSAL WOMAN

Menopause can happen in your forties or fifties, but the average age is fifty-one in the United States. Trust me, it gets easier to lose weight once menopause has finished and is much easier than for perimenopausal woman. Here, hormones are rapidly depleting and your body is looking for new ways of maintaining a proper weight and a new way of handling these hormonal changes.

While the hormonal changes of menopause might make you more likely to gain weight around your abdomen than around your hips and thighs, hormonal changes alone don't necessarily trigger menopausal weight gain. For example, muscle mass typically diminishes with age, while fat increases. Loss of muscle mass decreases the rate at which your body uses energy.

Estrogen appears to help control body weight in animal studies. With lower estrogen levels, lab animals tend to eat more and be less physically active. And though you're not a mouse. . . Reduced estrogen may also lower metabolism. The lack of estrogen causes one more thing: The body uses starches and blood sugar less effectively, which increases fat storage and makes it harder to lose weight.

Here is the protein booster shake recipe for menopausal and postmenopausal women:

Protein Booster Shake for the Menopausal or Postmenopausal Woman

3,000 mg L-leucine
750 mg L-valine
750 mg L-isoleucine
5,000 mg L-glutamine
1,000 mg L-carnitine
1 tablespoon macadamia nut oil
1 tablespoon freshly ground chia seeds
¼ cup unsweetened coconut or almond milk
6 ice cubes

Combine all the ingredients in a blender and puree until smooth.

A Note on the Ingredients

The difference here is the amount of glutamine and carnitine. These doses have been shown in studies to boost metabolism while maintaining muscle mass and shrinking fat cells.

THE YOUNG MAN

This is by far the easiest group to work with. The only things that get in the way are generally willpower and consistency. Young men have everything going for them when it comes to weight loss. They have excellent metabolisms, high testosterone levels, more lean muscle mass even if they are overweight or obese, and a body that naturally wants to be thin.

Having said that, we are entering into an era of unhealthy, overweight, metabolically challenged young men. There are probably many reasons this is taking place, the first and foremost being the abundance of fast food and junk food. Many young men who were physically active in sports in high school and college think that eating poorly is something they could always easily compensate for, so they get lulled into thinking they can eat anything they want. But that kind of eating quickly catches up to you when you start working, get married, and raise children. And then you don't know what to eat because you never learned in the first place.

The second reason—and the one for which there is no science yet to back me up, but trust me, there will be—is that men live in an estrogenized world. Phytoestrogens are estrogen-like substances that mimic the effects of estrogen in the body. I have seen a rash of younger men who have lower testosterone levels than their grandfathers. I can think of no other reason than the poisonous food supply and the levels of toxins, including endocrine disruptors (cleaning supplies, receipts, that new car smell, and many others). Any time you eat an animal injected with or fed growth hormones and antibiotics, chickens that are not fed earthworms and bugs, or any source of animal protein that doesn't graze on grass or fish that don't swim freely in the ocean, you are contributing to your lack of testosterone and your weight issues.

And just because your sex drive is good (which is the only thing you really care about as a young man), that doesn't mean you aren't suffering from low testosterone levels. You may be young, but you aren't invincible, and if you need to lose weight, the A-List Diet is the best place to start because it will provide you with the necessary amino acid protein shakes to get you back to where you want to be.

Here is the protein booster shake recipe for young men:

Protein Booster Shake for the Young Man

6,000 mg L-leucine
1,500 mg L-valine
1,500 mg L-isoleucine
8,000 mg L-glutamine
1 tablespoon macadamia nut oil
¼ cup unsweetened coconut or almond milk
6 ice cubes

Combine all the ingredients in a blender and puree until smooth.

A Note on the Ingredients

The difference in this shake is the larger amounts of the branched-chain amino acids. Young men need a larger dose of the building blocks to build and maintain muscle while losing weight.

THE ANDROPAUSAL MAN OVER FORTY

Yes, men get their own version of menopause. Just don't call it man-o-pause, please. Why do you think you have a mid-life crisis? It's your hormones, too.

Andropause is the result of a gradual decline in testosterone levels as men age. It is caused by the reduction of the hormones testosterone and dehydroepiandrosterone in middle-aged men. Testosterone assists the male body in building protein and is crucial for normal sex drive and stamina. Testosterone also contributes to several metabolic functions including bone formation, production of blood cells in the bone marrow, liver function, and, of course, erections.

When men get into their early thirties, they begin losing testosterone at a rate of 1 to 2 percent a year. A recent World Health Organization report analyzed male hormones and found that the testosterone levels in most seventy-year-old men were 10 percent of the level in males who are twenty-five years old. By the time men are between the ages of forty and fifty-five, they will likely begin experiencing symptoms of andropause. These include irritability, weight gain especially around the middle, sleep apnea, memory loss, diminished libido, hair loss, erectile dysfunction, depression, fatigue, and muscle loss.

Since testosterone is a key component in building protein, you will need more amino acids to take up the slack—which is why the protein booster shake for this group of men is the most potent of them all.

Here is the protein booster shake recipe for andropausal men:

Protein Booster Shake for the Andropausal Man over Forty

6,000 mg L-leucine
1,500 mg L-valine
1,500 mg L-isoleucine
10,000 mg L-glutamine
3,000 mg L-carnitine
1 tablespoon macadamia nut oil
1 teaspoon ground turmeric
¼ cup unsweetened coconut or almond milk
6 ice cubes

Combine all the ingredients in a blender and puree until smooth.

A Note on the Ingredients

The andropausal man needs high doses of the branched-chain amino acids in order to maintain and restore the loss of muscle mass. The high dose of glutamine is included for insulin resistance and the carnitine to aid in the conversion of fat to muscle. The turmeric is an anti-inflammatory companion because as those visceral fat cells die, they release toxins that are inflammatory in nature.

THE DIET-CHALLENGED MAN OR WOMAN

This is the dieter who has been on and off diets their entire life. This is the person who has tried every diet under the sun with varying degrees of success. As I mentioned earlier, it's possible to identify with multiple categories. For simplicity, resort to this category if you aren't having success with your first choice.

It is important to change up the foods you eat, rotate your protein sources, and get those all-important A-list protein booster shakes and protein boost shots (see chapter 5) so you can start losing weight again and never reach the plateau that always frustrates you and leads you to give up trying to lose weight.

Here is the protein booster shake for the diet challenged:

Protein Booster Shake for the Diet-Challenged Man or Woman

3,000 mg L-leucine
750 mg L-valine
750 mg L-isoleucine
5,000 mg L-glutamine
3,000 mg L-carnitine
1 tablespoon macadamia nut oil
1 tablespoon freshly ground chia seeds
1 tablespoon freshly ground flaxseed
1 teaspoon ground turmeric
¼ cup unsweetened coconut or almond milk
6 ice cubes

Combine all the ingredients in a blender and puree until smooth.

A Note on the Ingredients

As you can see, this shake is really a dose of all the ingredients from each of the other protein booster shakes. If all else fails, this will surely do the trick.

Marla's A-List Diet Story

Marla, a fifty-four-year-old woman, came to see me because she was at least a hundred pounds overweight. She was diabetic and was unable to control her blood sugar, so her doctor put her on insulin. Marla hated insulin and told me that she would do anything to get off it. She was okay with taking nutritional supplements and even her diabetes medications, but the thought of insulin scared her.

After doing all the necessary blood work, we started with the detox program (see chapter 3) and then the perimenopausal shake, along with two protein boost shots per day. Marla has lost eighty-six pounds as of this writing. She had been on many other diets over the years, but she told me the other day that the A-List Diet is the only one that has worked for this long—all the others either stopped working or she gave up. We both looked at each other and said, "Protein boosting!" She can't get enough of them. Marla is no longer on insulin and takes just one pill per day for her diabetes instead of six.

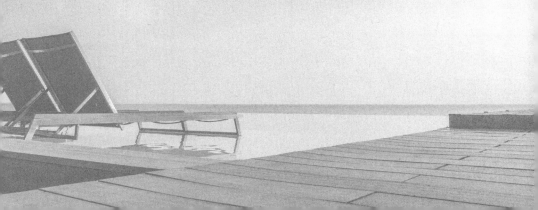

PHASE ONE
DETOX (WEEK ONE)

CHAPTER THREE

The A-List Detox

The A-List Diet consists of three phases:

1. The first phase, the detox phase, is for anyone who wants to get healthy. It lasts for a week.
2. The second phase focuses on the best weight-loss practices I have used to date. It lasts until you reach your goal weight.
3. The third phase is for those who don't need to lose weight— these folks just want to stay healthy and look and feel younger forever—and for those who have already reached their goal weight.

The detox phase is necessary to rid the bowels of the toxins that are stored there. A good detox also helps restore balance to your digestive tract, or microbiome. And it is becoming increasingly clear that the health of our microbiome is a major component to weight loss. It seems every day there is a new study that points out how certain bacteria in your gut, or lack thereof, could be contributing to your inability to lose weight or your inability to maintain your ideal weight.

Data shows that gut flora have a hand in your susceptibility to a long list of metabolic disorders. We're talking about some of the deadliest, most costly, and most prevalent illnesses plaguing our society. According to a recent study published in the journal *Nature*, subjects with a predominance of "bad" bacteria in their gut struggle with obesity, insulin resistance, dangerous lipid profiles, and higher levels of inflammation more often than individuals with a healthier microbiome.

MY PERSONAL DETOX MISSTEP

An effective detoxification strategy can transform your health in countless ways. And it's an important element to the A-List Diet. Just don't do what I did the first time I detoxed.

What I am about to tell you is going to sound drastic. (It was.) But I went on my first detox by accident when I was trying to lose weight as a teen. For Lent, I decided to give up food—yes, all food—for the entire forty days leading up to Easter.

My mother was horrified, obviously. And my grades in school suffered. Frankly, I was lucky I didn't wind up in the hospital. Still, I can't say that nothing good came out of it.

Let's be clear: I never should have gone without food for such a long time. But after the first few days, I have to admit, I felt amazing and had tons of energy. And when all was said and done, it accomplished what I wanted—which was sixty pounds gone.

Needless to say, my opinions on healthy detox practices have changed significantly since then. For one thing, I would never want you to follow in my teenage footsteps. Unfortunately, I'm sure many misguided people take such drastic measures. And that's why I think it's high time we talked about the right way to deal with stored-up toxins in your body.

Patients ask me about this subject constantly. And if they're asking, then I am sure you're wondering about it, too. So, with that introduction and my requisite cautionary tale out of the way, let's dive right into the details.

THE A-LIST DETOX

First things first: The detox phase is only seven days.

That week may seem like an eternity now, but trust me, the time goes by incredibly quickly. You will be feeling so much better that by the end of day seven, you might not want to stop—but you must stop and move on to the next phase (details to follow). The detox itself is really simple—there's no fancy equipment or elaborate planning involved. Just a quality detox supplement and a multivitamin, along with the specific liquids and foods listed for each of the seven days (in unlimited quantities).

The only other two products I would recommend during this phase are Dr. Ohhira's Probiotics and a supplement called Reg'Activ Detox & Liver Health, which helps your body produce the antioxidant glutathione. Glutathione is a very important aid in detoxification, but in my opinion, oral glutathione supplements can't be absorbed. Reg'Activ contains the probiotic *Lactobacillus fermentum* ME-3, which clinical research shows can help the body synthesize glutathione naturally. In other words, Reg'Activ is able to extract glutathione from its surrounding environment and recycle spent glutathione back into its active form. There is no other supplement like it on the market yet.

As for any other nutritional supplements you may be taking, I recommend stopping them for this week. Personally, I like to give my body a break from nutritional supplements every once in a while. The perfect time to do that is during a detox. This break allows your body to focus solely on the work of eliminating the toxins from your system. Once you're done, you can—and should—resume your normal supplement regimen along with the new ones that I will be outlining specifically for the A-list program and, of course, the all-important protein-boosting shakes and shots.

However, you should continue with any medications you may be taking. It's never a good idea to stop taking a medication abruptly.

And, of course, you should talk to your doctor before starting this or any detox regimen. (But be forewarned: Most mainstream physicians aren't likely to have the first clue about detoxing. So don't expect much in the way of supportive feedback. It's probably best to work with a holistic physician, a naturopathic physician, or a certified clinical nutritionist if you're undertaking any serious detox regimen.)

I should also be clear that pregnant or lactating women should not do this cleanse. Neither should children or anyone with a truly debilitating disease that isn't well controlled. If you are diabetic or on high blood pressure medications, there is a strong likelihood that you will need to take less of these particular medications, during and after the detox. If you fall into this category, you truly must discuss this phase of the diet with your personal physician. If you do not have an open-minded personal physician who can guide you, I strongly recommend starting with phase two, which begins in the next chapter, and eliminating the detox phase altogether.

But, quite frankly, anyone else can benefit from a thorough detox. It's the perfect remedy for my patients who are looking to jump-start their weight loss programs and for those who have been stuck in a cycle of yo-yo dieting.

Even for people who just want to "clean house"—especially if you're regularly exposed to chemical solvents by profession, or perhaps from frequent trips to the nail salon—the strategy I'm about to share can be a life-changer.

SAFE, EFFECTIVE DETOX
IS A THREE-STEP PROCESS

The first stage of detoxification is to modify toxins into substances that are water soluble so they are more readily excreted from the body. Your body naturally contains a family of enzymes specifically designed for this process called cytochrome P450. They reside in the membranes of healthy liver cells.

Stage one is necessary since fat-soluble toxins can't be cleared out of your body without it. Fat-soluble toxins can be stored in every organ in your body, including the liver, kidneys, skin, and, most importantly for our purposes, fat cells. But this stage can also be dangerous. That's because the intermediary end products of stage one of detoxification are often more harmful than the toxins from which they were created.

This is why stage two of the detox phase is so critically important. Stage two is called conjugation. And it's exactly what it sounds like. Compounds, like glutathione or amino acids, join, or conjugate, with water-soluble toxins to neutralize them and prepare them for excretion.

All this is in preparation for stage three, which is called elimination. This is also exactly what it sounds like. The neutralized, conjugated toxins are safely eliminated from your body through your urine, bile, and bowel movements.

HERE'S HOW

On days one and two of the A-list detox, I recommend that you drink only pure water and/or herbal teas consistently throughout the day. For tea, it must be plain: no sugar, sugar substitute, or milk/creamer of any kind. It may seem meager, but I promise if you are anything like my patients or myself, you will not feel hungry.

After the first two days, nutritious broths can be added to your diet. I highly encourage you to make your own bone broths. They are the simplest things to make, but as with any recipe, the better your ingredients, the tastier and more nutritious the dish.

On day four, you add eggs to the menu. Why eggs? Well, they're nature's purest form of protein. But it is crucial to buy not only organic eggs but eggs from free-range hens raised outside in a pasture on grass, eating earthworms and bugs. Not from hens crammed into cages, fed "enriched" omega-3 corn, along with hefty servings of hormones and antibiotics. Free-range hens produce eggs that have the nutritional profile nature intended, with an omega-3 to omega-6 ratio of 1:1.

On day five, you get to add avocado. Another perfect food, one that is rich in monounsaturated fatty acids. It is almost 100 percent omega-9 fat. Omega-9 fats are neutral fats, which mean they do not cause inflammation in any way. They are also the fat that is the heart healthiest and the best for our skin. Monos have been shown to boost your metabolism, and that's why they make an appearance on day five.

Next up to introduce is nuts on day six. Any nut will do (keeping in mind that peanuts are a legume and not a nut), but I prefer pistachios, macadamia nuts, walnuts, and almonds. The healthiest option for any nut is unsalted and raw. However, roasted and/or salted work just as well. Macadamia nuts are an incredible source of the monounsaturated omega-9 fatty acid. Almonds are the clear winner in the omega-3 anti-inflammatory category, and pistachios—while much maligned—are surprisingly high in monounsaturated omega-9 fats and are packed with minerals like copper, manganese, iron, magnesium, zinc, and selenium, as well as many of the B vitamins. They're a wonderful way to get the cofactors your body needs to help in detoxification.

And last but not least, we begin to add some light, flaky fish, such as cod or halibut, on day seven. The fish should be wild, low on the food chain so as to decrease the likelihood of mercury contamination, and as fresh as you can afford.

The A-list detox is a perfect cleanse without the unnecessary and unscientifically proven need to starve yourself with fruit juices for weeks on end. (And fruit juices, by the way, are all sugar. And as you know by now, sugar is a killer.)

But please, no matter what you do, don't forget to drink water. It is essential to stay hydrated. When your body is preparing for all those toxins to be eliminated, you need enough water to allow that to happen. Elimination of the toxins is key or you run the risk of them moving to a different part of your body and causing more damage.

So again, *drink a lot of water.* A good rule of thumb is to divide your weight by half and drink that amount in ounces of water—more if you are going to exercise.

THE DETOX SCIENCE

Let's quickly review the science behind all this. There are five processes that must occur in stages one and two of the detox, and each one has a specific purpose in what it will help remove from the body:

1. Sulfation
2. Glucuronidation
3. Acetylation
4. Amino acid conjugation (See what I mean? Almost every bodily function requires amino acids. The ones used for liver detox are glycine, taurine, and glutamine.)
5. Methylation

Each of those processes requires vitamin support to ensure proper detoxification. Just to name a few: vitamin C, alpha-lipoid acid, methionine, vitamin B_{12}, folic acid, choline, and magnesium. I know most conventional doctors think that vitamins will just make your urine expensive. While that may be true in a sense, we simply can't get the amount of nutrients from the food we eat, so you will need a good quality multivitamin (something like my MetaMulti Advanced formula). And the next time you get the expensive urine line, kindly remind your doctor that most drugs are eliminated through the kidneys, and if you are on any prescription medication, I can ensure you that your urine is already quite expensive.

THE DETOX SUPPLEMENTS

I used to recommend—and follow—a simple water fast for detoxification. It worked well for me and my most dedicated clients, but I knew there had to be a better way to detox. That's when I came across literature that supported the A-list detox that I've outlined for you to follow. It's one thing to detox; it's another to keep your metabolism at full capacity while doing so.

And science shows that supporting your body's natural elimination processes along will yield better, faster results. Which is why the market has exploded with all sorts of detox supplements.

So how do you choose the right one?

A good detox product will include ingredients that support all three of the critical detox steps I outlined above. Unfortunately, many of the ones you'll find on the shelves of your local supplement shop don't offer complete support. And since detox is such an important part of both achieving good health and maintaining it, I wanted to be able to offer my patients a product they—and I—could trust. So I formulated my own. I call it DetoxLogic. Obviously, you don't need to get the product that I've developed, but if you don't, I would recommend that you at least look at all the ingredients and get one that is as similar to it as you can.

I made sure DetoxLogic has everything you need to make your detox as efficient and effective as possible. And the first thing it needed was reliable liver support. Milk thistle is typically the go-to herb for liver support. But it's important to make sure it contains enough of one particular compound, silymarin. Volumes of research support silymarin's ability to protect your liver on the cellular level, boosting both membrane stability and antioxidant defense.

I included an ultra-bioavailable, patented form of silymarin called Siliphos in DetoxLogic. And I was also able to find ultra-bioavailable forms of grapeseed extract and curcumin to add as well. Both of these ingredients offer additional antioxidant support, which is critical to help keep free radical byproducts from step one of detoxification in check. Curcumin also plays double-duty by helping promote bile flow.

DetoxLogic also includes a comprehensive dose of conjugating amino acids to help bind toxins. But I also added another unique ingredient—a green algae called broken cell wall chlorella, noted for its ability to bind with heavy metals. Please note that this is not a heavy metal detox. A heavy metal detox is a form of chelation where we eliminate toxic metal burdens such as mercury and lead that may have accumulated over the years from pollution, leaded gasoline, eating too much fish, or even dental fillings. That is a different process than what we are trying to achieve with DetoxLogic.

Last, but certainly not least, my detox formula needed to offer targeted elimination support. And that starts with probiotics and prebiotics, which are food for all that good bacteria. DetoxLogic includes five billion colony-forming units (CFUs) of gut-strengthening *Bacillus coagulans* and burdock—an abundant source of the prebiotic inulin. I also added two more herbs to the DetoxLogic—uva ursi leaf and stinging nettle—to help your urinary tract and kidneys flush out metabolic waste.

A proper detox is a wonderful opportunity to take charge of your health and make those changes you want to see happen. Who buys your food? Who prepares your food? Who orders your food? You do! And it's just as easy to have the foods that will help you achieve your goals around you as those that won't. Don't be a victim in this situation. Stop letting being overweight happen to you. You chose what to eat before, and now you can choose other, more improved, and certainly healthier things to eat. I think being in charge of what you eat can be so empowering. Food is truly one of those things that you are in total control of. So use that power for good and not for evil.

I think our relationship to food is so highly emotionally charged that I wrote an entire book about it, called *Thin for Good*. If you are a very emotional eater, that book would make a good companion to this book.

THE A-LIST DETOX PROTOCOL REVIEW

I've been using this detox protocol in my practice for the past couple of years. And my only regret is not developing it sooner.

My patients have been reporting all sorts of benefits. Everything from more energy and vitality to weight loss and even improved sleep. But perhaps most importantly, patients who detox experience significant decreases in inflammation—something that, as I've mentioned many times already in this book, affects every single part of your body in a very serious way.

Best of all, there are no real side effects with this detox. Some patients have experienced a little diarrhea at the beginning. Some get constipated (which isn't really constipation at all, simply a smaller bulk of stool as the week progresses). But both are perfectly normal and safe.

Bottom line, this program has a lot of unique components that you won't find in any other detox plan, product, or formulation. But the proof is in the pudding. So let me share a quick patient story with you.

A year or so ago, I saw a patient who had visited a number of doctors, both conventional and integrative, for help with her persistent pain and fatigue. I'd been treating her for about a year with some success. But I decided she would be one of my first patients to try this new detox protocol. (I always figure that if something will help my most difficult cases, it will help almost anyone.)

To make a long story short, by the time she finished this detox, she looked like a whole new person. She'd lost eight pounds. The color had returned to her face. And she was even talking about going back to work—something that she thought she'd have to give up forever. And that was in just one week.

You just can't argue with results like that.

So let's go over the A-list detox one more time for good measure:

Days One and Two	pure water and/or herbal teas drunk consistently throughout the day so as to not get dehydrated or hungry (for tea, plain only: no sugar, sugar substitute, or milk/creamer of any kind)
Day Three	water, herbal teas, and other clear liquids, including broths
Day Four	liquids, broths, and eggs
Day Five	liquids, broths, eggs, and avocado
Day Six	liquids, broths, eggs, avocado, and nuts
Day Seven	liquids, broths, eggs, avocado, nuts, and simply cooked fish

1. Consume as much as you desire of these foods and liquids each day.
2. Drink plenty of liquids even on the days you begin to eat foods. A good rule of thumb is to divide your body weight by half and drink that amount in ounces per day.
3. Take a good multivitamin—my favorite is one that I formulated specifically for the A-List Diet called MetaMulti Advanced. Take two capsules three times per day.
4. Take a good detox supplement formula. Again, my favorite is the product I developed specifically for the A-List Diet called DetoxLogic. Take two pills three times per day.
5. Take one Dr. Ohhira's Probiotics capsule twice per day.
6. Take one Reg'Activ capsule twice per day.

The detox is the part of the diet that A-listers like the best because the results are quick and easy. That said, Mike, a rap icon, almost cried when I explained to him that he wouldn't be eating for two days. I never expected such behavior from such a macho guy—he literally sat in my office for half an hour complaining about how he wouldn't be able to go that long without food. I reminded him that the Grammys were two weeks away and he would be very shirtless on stage. He dug deep, did it, and called me on day three to tell me that he was amazed that he was never hungry at all. By day seven he had lost ten pounds. He was a happy man.

You can expect results like this, but please don't be discouraged if you don't lose quite that much. You will lose weight and feel better and that's our main goal. The A-List Diet is designed to help anyone achieve the weight loss or weight management goals they desire while not feeling hungry or deprived. You will learn how to eat healthy foods that turn on your metabolism without starving you. Now that you are detoxed and your liver is clean and your metabolism is revving, let the real work begin.

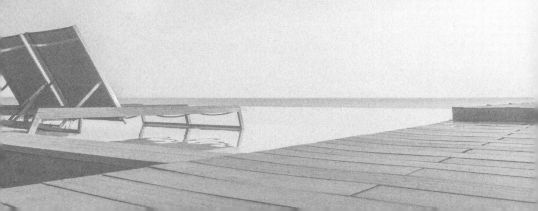

PHASE TWO

THE A-LIST
WEIGHT LOSS
EATING PROGRAM
(WEEK TWO AND BEYOND)

CHAPTER FOUR

Food Recommendations

A fter the detox week, you will be on a regular A-list weight loss eating program. Your weight loss now will average one to three pounds per week (or sometimes less). Don't get discouraged if and when things slow down. It is a slow and steady weight loss that allows your body to lose fat rather than water weight. The point of this process is to become healthy and lose weight, neither of which has to happen overnight.

The A-List Diet is built upon the principles of eating the foods that support health and weight management, balancing hormones, and decreasing inflammation in any way we can. Balancing the correct proteins for your dieting type, choosing the optimal fats and vegetables, and protein boosting go a long way in helping you manage your weight issues.

Now that you've been thoroughly detoxed, the fun begins because you get to eat food. Remember the six types of A-list dieters from chapter 2? Just as the amino acid contents vary for the protein booster shakes depending on your type, there are some foods that I recommend dieters in each group eat more of. Everyone needs all the amino acids but, according to the type of dieter you are, you will need different proportions of certain ones—the key A-list differentiation from any other diet program out there today. The following outline will help you achieve those goals since these particular foods contain more of what your body requires. You don't need to worry about this list if you follow my menu plan, but this guide is most helpful when eating out or grocery shopping.

1. **Perimenopausal women:** Be sure to include in your diet orange roughy, pike, cod, kelp, wakame, cauliflower, garlic, avocado, kale, kohlrabi, cucumbers, Brazil nuts, and sunflower seeds.
2. **Women in their twenties and thirties:** Be sure to include in your diet grass-fed, lean beef, fatty fish such as salmon and tuna, halibut, cucumbers, white mushrooms, and pumpkin seeds.
3. **Menopausal or postmenopausal women:** Be sure to include in your diet all types of fish (particularly pike, which has more of certain aminos for this group of women), lamb, eggs, nuts, watercress, fennel, endive, kale, broccoli rabe, asparagus, and swamp cabbage.
4. **Young men:** Be sure to include in your diet pork, turkey breast, bison, collard greens, mustard greens, kale, and peanut butter.
5. **Andropausal men over forty:** Be sure to include in your diet lean pork, grass-fed beef, buffalo, turkey breast, pike, scallops, parsley, okra, and asparagus.
6. **The diet challenged:** Be sure to include in your diet shrimp, scallops, mussels, sardines, salmon, turkey breast, bone broth, eggs, seaweed, bok choy, leafy greens, spinach, okra, and asparagus.

I have found that while some people just want to be told what to eat, long-term success comes from making healthy choices. We eat at all sorts of places where we can't always get what we want or know what to expect. That's where these lists come in handy. One trick I learned from my patients is that they actually take photos of healthy foods and photos of the lists and keep these photos on their phones so they always know what to choose—that's an A-list tip!

At the end of the book, I've included menu plans for thirty days of phase two. Although you may be dieting for longer than four weeks, a thirty-day plan should be enough to get you on the right path toward your ultimate weight goal. But at any time, you can simply choose foods from the following lists and enjoy!

PROTEINS

chicken	Cornish game hen	duck	goose
guinea hen	pheasant	beef	pork
lamb	veal	rabbit	emu
venison	frog	goat	mutton
ostrich	rabbit	antelope	boar
bison	alligator	grouse	liver
beef kidney	tripe	tongue	sweetbreads
jerky	monkfish	blackfish	grouper
cobra	shark	dolphin	mahi-mahi
marlin	lemonfish	striped bass	cod
scrod	John Dory	yellow fish	red fish
white sea bass	kingfish	flounder	halibut
sand dabs	sole	mullets	perch
wall-eyed pike	porgy	sea bream	red snapper
rockfish	blue snapper	orange roughy	tilefish
tuna	eel	anchovies	catfish
skipjack	sturgeon	arctic char	black cod (sablefish)
bluefish	buffalo fish	butterfish	salmon
herring	sardines	shad	sea trout
smelt	Spanish mackerel	rainbow trout	whitefish
bacalao (salted cod)	abalone	clam	scallops

Continued on next page . . .

"Proteins" continued . . .

calamari	cockles	conch	crab
crawfish	cuttlefish	langoustine	mussels
shrimp	lobster	octopus	oysters
periwinkle	snails	sea cucumber	prawns
squid	whelk	caviar	roe
eggs	soy protein	texturized vegetable protein	tempeh
seitan	nori	wakame	kombu
dulse	arame	duck eggs	quail eggs
salted duck eggs	thousand-year eggs	ostrich eggs	

As for quantities of the above-named foods, there really are no limits. Simply choose more from the foods that are recommended for your dieter type from the lists outlined above and always refer to the alkaline list in chapter 6. But don't go overboard. You need to eat protein, but it should be spread out over each meal. The A-listers don't ever go hungry, so you will likely eat less than before because you will be more satisfied with the foods you are eating, and they will keep you fuller longer. Shoot for about 1 gram of protein per pound of body weight per day—somewhat less if you are female and somewhat more if you are male.

COMPLEX CARBOHYDRATES: VEGETABLES

watercress	fennel	purslane	kale
spinach	snap peas (technically a legume)	artichokes	asparagus
Swiss chard	green beans	radishes	celery
cabbage	broccoli sprouts	broccoli rabe	collard greens

parsley	mustard greens	broccoli	baby zucchini (courgettes)
garden cress	beet greens	cauliflower	pak choi
arugula	Brussels sprouts	bamboo shoots	taro leaf or callaloo
alfalfa sprouts	turnip greens	kohlrabi	okra
chicory	dandelion greens	escarole	swamp cabbage
Chinese cabbage	bok choy	avocado	broccoflower
broccolini	broccoli romanesco	bitter melon or balsam pear	Chinese okra
fuzzy melon	Indian bitter melon	opo squash	buckwheat sprouts
daikon sprouts	fenugreek sprouts	mung bean spouts	onion sprouts
radish sprouts	snow pea shoots	celtuce	Chinese broccoli
Chinese spinach	chrysanthemum leaves	kai choy	jute leaf
jam leaf	pumpkin greens	endive	Bibb lettuce
Boston lettuce	chicory	mâche	red endive
frisée	green leaf lettuce	red leaf lettuce	iceberg lettuce
lollo rosso	mizuna	oak leaf lettuce	radicchio
red mustard greens	romaine lettuce	tatsoi	eggplant
spaghetti squash	globe squash	pattypan squash	scallopini squash
tinda	yellow squash	zucchini	cucumber
red bell pepper	green bell pepper	Cubanelle	pimento
Anaheim chile	ancho chile	poblano chile	banana pepper
cherry pepper	Thai chile	cayenne pepper	chilaca
jalapeño pepper	serrano chile	Fresno chile	habanero pepper
Holland chile	manzana chile	mirasol chile	New Mexico green chile
Scotch bonnet chile	rocoto chile	serrano pepper	shishito chile

Continued on next page . . .

"Complex Carbohydrates: Vegetables" continued . . .

yellow wax pepper	cascabel chile	catarina chile	red chile
chipotle pepper	guajillo chile	mulato chile	sequin pepper
puya chile	olives	capers	tomatillos
cardoon	Chinese celery	fiddlehead fern	hearts of palm
rhubarb	white asparagus	wild asparagus	green onion
leek	ramp	spring onion	Bermuda onion
white onion	cipollini onion	pearl onion	red onion
shallot	yellow onion	garlic	elephant garlic
garlic greens	Thai ginger	Chinese ginger	ginger root
green ginger	myoga ginger	turmeric	green cabbage
red cabbage	napa cabbage	savoy cabbage	su hoy
yau choy	string beans	yard-long bean	winged bean
Chinese long bean	dragon tongue bean	French bean	Italian flat bean
sator beans	wax bean	chives	guacamole
abalone cap mushroom	black trumpet mushroom	blewit mushroom	button mushroom
cauliflower mushroom	chanterelle	chestnut mushroom	hen of the woods mushrooms
cinnamon cap mushroom	clamshell mushroom	cremini mushroom	enoki mushrooms
gamboni mushroom	maitake mushroom	matsutake mushroom	morels
oyster mushroom	portobello mushrooms	shiitake mushroom	shimeji mushroom
trumpet mushroom	truffles	no pale	nopalitos
sauerkraut	pickles	rhubarb	cornichons
kimchi	pepperoncini	shiritaki noodle	borage flower
chive flowers	chamomile	chrysanthemums	geraniums
hibiscus flowers	golden needles	impatiens	lavender
lemon blossoms	mimosa blossoms	nasturtium	orange blossom
pansy	sage blossoms	squash blossoms	

While not in alphabetical order, the vegetables toward the top are more of the "superfoods." I advise incorporating more of these into your diet. Any vegetable will do as long as it is from this list. Again, you really can eat as much of this list of foods as you would like. They are filling and nutritious—all A-listers can't go wrong with vegetables.

DAIRY

heavy cream	clotted cream	Devonshire cream	crema
crème fraîche	clabber cream	kaymak	kashk
qurut	smetana	sour cream	almond milk
coconut butter	coconut milk	rice milk	hemp milk
soy milk	cashew milk	Boursin	Rondelé
Alouette	buttermilk cheese	caprini	chaka
chèvre or goat cheese	cottage cheese	cream cheese	farmer cheese
queso fresco	queso blanco	queso panela	queso para freír
Gervais	pot cheese	paneer	kefir cheese
mascarpone	mizithra	Neufchâtel	queso de matarte
requesón	ricotta	robiola piemonte	whey cheeses
yogurt cheese	boursault	Brie	Brillat-Savarin
Brinza	camembert	caprice des dieux	Carré de l'Est
chaource	coulommiers	Crema Danica	Crescenza
epoisses	excelsior	Explorateur	feta
handkäse	harz	Humboldt Fog	kochkaese
Liederkranz	livarot	mainz	manouri
Maroilles	morbier	paglietta	Pont-l'Évêque
Reblochon	ricotta salata	Robiola	Schloss
Saint-André	Saint-Marcellin	stracchino	Teleme
asadero	beaumont	Bierkäse	Bel Paese

Continued on next page . . .

"Dairy" continued . . .

brick cheese	buffalo milk mozzarella	caciocavallo	California Jack
casero	chaubier	corsu vecchiu	esrom
fiore sardo	Gouda	Haloumi	Havarti
Jack	lager kase	laguiole	lappi
Limburger	mozzarella	Munster	oka
Ossau-Iraty	Port-Salut	provolone	queso menonita
Saint-Paulin	samsoe	scamorza	string cheese
Syrian cheese	taleggio	tilsit	Tomme Crayeuse
Tomme de Savoie	Tybo	urgelia	Vacherin
abondance	Appenzeller	Asiago	Beaufort
caciotta	caerphilly	cantal	Cheddar
Cheshire	Colby	Comté	coon
Danbo	Derby	Edam	Emmentaler
Fontina	gamonedo	gjetost	Gloucester
graviera	greve	Gruyère	idiazabal
Jarlsberg	kashkaval	kasseri	Lancashire
leerdammer	red leicester	leyden	Mahón
manchego	mysost	nokkelost	primost
Raclette	Saint Nectaire	Swiss	Tête de Moine
queso añejo	grana padano	kefalotyri	mimolette
Parmesan	pecorino	queso enchilada	saenkanter
sapsago	bleu cheese	Bavarian blue	Bleu d'Auvergne
Bleu de Bresse	Bleu des Causses	bleu de chèvre	bleu de gex
blue castello	cables	cambozola	Irish cashel
Danish blue	Fourme d'Ambert	Gorgonzola	Maytag blue
Montbriac	picon	Roquefort	Saga blue
Saint Agur	Shropshire blue	Stilton	Valdeon
Västerbotten	Wensleydale	yak cheese	

As far as yogurt goes, it is made from milk, which has sugar in it. Even the unsweetened versions by their very nature have sugar, so it's really best to skip it altogether.

You should limit the creams to no more than 2 tablespoons per day.

Any nondairy milks or creams should be unsweetened and have no more than 4 grams of sugar per serving, and you should limit to one serving per day.

You should have no more than 2 ounces of cheese per day. The cheeses are listed in order: fresh, soft, semi-soft, semi-firm, firm, blue, and others. I ask that you stay away from processed cheese food products such as American cheese or Velveeta. As you can see, there are many cheeses you can choose from. The A-listers love variety.

NUTS AND NUT BUTTERS

almond	beechnut	black walnut	Brazil nut
butternut	candlenut	cashew	Chinese almond
filbert	hazelnut	coconut meat	hickory nut
macadamia nut	paradise nut	peanut (yes, it's a legume)	pecan
persona walnut	pine nut	pili nut	pistachio
walnut	white sesame seed	black sesame seed	pumpkin seed
sunflower seed	flaxseed	chia seed	hemp seed
egusi seed	hemp seed	psyllium seed	squash seed
watermelon seed			

No matter what kind of nut you choose, you really can't go wrong—they're all good. It's a proven fact that people who eat more nuts have a lower risk of metabolic syndrome. Plus, nuts are full of fiber, protein, iron, zinc, B vitamins, and other nutrients. They help protect your heart, lower blood pressure, reduce inflammation, and keep you feeling full. But there is just one small catch—it's easy to overdo it. So make sure you're not eating more than twenty nuts per day. Most of these nuts also come as nut butters. Limit that to 1½ tablespoons per day. (Please note that marzipan, although made from almonds, does have sugar, so that is not permitted for A-listers.)

And to be clear, you may have one or the other—not both. In other words, don't eat twenty nuts in the morning and then 1½ tablespoons of a nut butter in the afternoon. If you want to incorporate both into your daily diet, have less of each.

FRUITS

bilberry	blackberry	blueberry	boysenberry
cranberries	dew berry	frais des bois	golden raspberry
gooseberry	huckleberry	juneberry	keriberry
lingonberry	loganberry	raspberry	strawberry
ambrosia melon	canary melon	cantaloupe	casaba melon
Charentais melon	crane melon	Crenshaw melon	Galia melon
honeyball melon	honeydew melon	kharbouza melon	kiwano melon
ogen melon	Persian melon	Santa Claus melon	Sharlyn melon
Spanish melon	watermelon	yellow melon	balsam pear
feijoa	longan	litchi	rose apple
langsat	persimmon	starfruit	plumcot
plum	crabapple	passion fruit	acerola
tamarind	guava	buddha's hand citron	kumquat
Seville orange	lime	calamansi lime	Florida key lime
kaffir lime	kabosu lime	limequat	tamarillo
clementine	lemon	Meyer lemon	

These fruits have the lowest sugar content or are low on the glycemic index, so they won't significantly impact your blood sugar—or your waistline. You can enjoy ½ cup of fruits three times per week.

HERBS AND SPICES

file powder	cilantro	mint	baobab leaves
kuka	anise basil	bai-toey	betel leaf
chile leaf	garlic chives	flowering chives	holy basil
bay leaf	kaffir lime leaf	laksa leaf	la-lot leaf
lemon basil	lemongrass	licorice basil	Italian basil
mitsuba	ngo om	saw leaf herb	screw pine leaf
sesame leaf	perilla	sweet basil	yellow Chinese chives
angelica	bergamot	borage	chervil
chives	cicely	curly parsley	dill leaf
hyssop	Italian parsley	lemon balm	lemon thyme
lemon verbena	lovage	marjoram	opal basil
oregano	parsley	rosemary	sage
savory	summer savory	tarragon	thyme
winter savory	caraway seeds	celery seed	fenugreek seed
fennel seed	radish seed	avocado leaves	boldo leaves
culantro	epazote	guajes	hoja santa leaves
huauzontle	saffron	papalo	pepicha
romeritos	yerba buena	curry leaf	fenugreek leaves
turmeric leaves	jute	anise seed	alfalfa seed
allspice	cardamom	Chinese cinnamon	cinnamon
cloves	coriander seeds	cumin	dill seed

Continued on next page . . .

"Herbs and Spices" continued . . .

mace	dill seeds	mustard seed	dry mustard
poppy seeds	turmeric	vanilla bean	yellow mustard seed
black pepper	green pepper	pink pepper	white pepper
guinea pepper	malagueta pepper	osho sho	ukpo
Szechuan peppercorn	long pepper	star anise	Oriental Five Spice
caraway seeds	celery seed	ginger	lemon peel
nutmeg	orange peel	paprika	smoked paprika
achiote seed	cayenne pepper	red pepper flakes	red chile powder
pallilo	ajwain	amchoor	asafetida
black cumin	black mustard seeds	brown cardamom	brown mustard seeds
fenugreek	nigella	Aleppo pepper	mahlab
berbere	ras el hanout	celery salt	chili powder
lemon pepper	Old Bay	onion salt	onion powder
garlic salt	garlic powder	garlic	poultry seasoning
pickling spice	creole spice mix	salt	shichimi togarashi
beau monde	bouquet garni	fines herbes	herbes de Provence
quatre epices	chervil	cloves	rosemary
ehuru	marjoram	garam masala	menudo mix
taco seasoning	chat masala	curry powder	panch phoron
tandoori seasoning	kelp powder	baharat	zahter
hawaij	coriander	kosher salt	sea salt
bamboo salt	black salt	butter salt	coarse salt
French sea salt	Hawaiian salt	pretzel salt	extracts for cooking

Generally, there isn't a spice or herb in the world that isn't allowed on the A-list protocols. They add amazing variety to the foods you are eating and are a wonderful way to avoid diet boredom. Don't be afraid to try some of the things on the list you have never heard of. Some you will like, while others you will hate me for suggesting. But you won't know until you try. However, there are a few things to be careful of in the spice section. Most combination spices contain sugar even if it's not listed on the label. There are many foods in this country where sugar doesn't have to be listed on the label and spice mixes are one example. Steer clear of those and make your own spice mixes.

CONDIMENTS

harissa	creole mustard	whole grain mustard	Dijon mustard
hot mustard	Tabasco	Pickapeppa	Louisiana hot sauce
sriracha	relish	mayonnaise	Asian barbecue sauce
Asian chili paste	chee hou sauce	chili paste	fish sauce
hot chili sauce	soy sauce	tamari	green curry paste
hot garlic sauce	wasabi	nam prik pao	nuoc mam
nuoc cham	red curry paste	sambal bajak	sambal belacan
sambal dato lilang	sambal manis	sambal oelek	shrimp paste
toi sauce	yellow curry paste	aioli	anchovy paste
hollandaise sauce	horseradish	mint sauce	piccalilli
piri-piri sauce	tapenade	adobo sauce	chili verde
guacamole	pipian	recaito	red chile sauce
rocoto sauce	salsa verde	hummus	pesto
tahini			

These can generally be used with abandon. Feel free to explore this list, and note that hummus is here as a condiment and not meant to be eaten as a bowlful. Please limit hummus to 2 tablespoons per day.

FATS AND OILS

butter	clarified butter	ghee	caul fat
duck fat	goose fat	lard	goat butter
lardo	suet	avocado oil	bacon grease
hot chili oil	mustard oil	olive oil	macadamia nut oil
schmaltz			

Since I wrote an entire book on the subject of healthy oils, you can refer to *The Hamptons Diet* for full details. My preference remains macadamia nut oil or avocado oil for high-heat purposes and olive oil for cold uses only. Try to limit this category of food to 2 tablespoons per day, but that isn't a hard and fast rule. Personally, I use these foods with abandon. Just use the healthiest versions of this category that you can afford. And by all means, never use margarine, vegetable shortening, canola oil, or any imitation butter or butter-flavored sprays. (If you like to use cooking spray, buy a reusable spray bottle and put your own healthy oil in it.)

SWEETENERS

There are two sweeteners to use: stevia and lo han. Both are made from plants, both have no calories, and both can be used to your heart's content. While artificial sweeteners aren't allowed on the A-list program, they usually will not affect your weight loss. They just aren't healthy for you.

MISCELLANEOUS

unsweetened cocoa powder	gelatin	acidulated water	balsamic vinegar
apple cider vinegar	champagne vinegar	Chinese black vinegar	coconut vinegar

infused vinegar	herb vinegar	malt vinegar	palm vinegar
red rice vinegar	red wine vinegar	rice vinegar	tarragon vinegar
umeboshi vinegar	white rice vinegar	white vinegar	white wine vinegar

There is no limit as to the amount of these foods that you may eat.

DRINKS

coffee	tea	herbal tea	water
club soda	sparkling water	seltzer water	sparkling mineral water
flat mineral water	flavored unsweetened water	clam juice	lemon juice
lime juice			

The water should come in glass bottles. The teas and coffee should be organic and water processed. You can have as much of this category as you like, and you should take your weight, divide it by half, and drink that much water in ounces each day. When exercising, you should drink about 8 ounces every fifteen minutes to maintain proper hydration.

ALCOHOL

aquavit	amber rum	batavia arrack	blended whiskey
bourbon	Canadian whiskey	corn whiskey	white rum
gin	grain alcohol	Irish whiskey	mescal
poteen	pulque	rye whiskey	Scotch whiskey
sour mash whiskey	tequila	vodka	whiskey
bitters			

Alcohol should be drunk with caution as the jury is still out as to how much is a healthy amount to be consuming per week. Currently, the thinking is as follows: For men, 210 milliliters of alcohol per week with no more than 40 milliliters at one time and with two alcohol-free days per week. For women, 140 milliliters of alcohol per week with no more than 30 milliliters at a time and with two alcohol-free days per week. Further, alcohol should never be combined with mixers that have sugar, like tonic water. If you choose a mixer, stick to water or club soda. Obviously, if you want the most effect from the diet, I would avoid alcohol altogether or stick to clear liquors.

THE A-LIST ANSWERS TO COMMON DIETING QUESTIONS

There are a couple of things that all my patients ask or that will inevitably come up during an interview, and I would like to address them before you get started on your new A-list journey.

1. **What's the best ratio of protein to fats to carbs?** This is always a tough question, because I think that the ideal foods to eat are those that are high quality that contain phytonutrients, antioxidants, and the correct fatty acids. They should be nutrient dense, slow down the insulin response in the body and allow the body to heal, slow down the aging process, repair cells, and repair the effects of inflammation, or at the very least reduce it. Low-quality foods such as processed foods or nonorganic foods are more important to be avoided than a simple ratio of macronutrients. That being said, when push comes to shove, the ideal diet to me is generally 30 to 35 percent from protein, 30 to 35 percent from fat, and the rest from carbohydrates such as vegetables, and some fruit. Just having one serving of vegetables per day reduces your risk of death

by 16 percent. Consuming five servings of vegetables per day reduces your risk of death by 42 percent.

2. **Should I count calories?** The short answer, once again, is *no!* There is a clear-cut distinction between a healthy, nutritive calorie and a non-nutritive calorie. And this is where most commercial diet programs get it all wrong. In order for you to have meaningful weight loss and a successful weight management program, you must understand why certain foods are healthy and contribute to your body functioning well and others don't. Programs that focus on calories miss the entire point of eating to be healthy, so weight loss (and, more importantly, weight management) suffers as a result. So, what happens in this scenario is, "I will have 100 calories of ice cream instead of broccoli, and that's the same thing." No! The way your body responds to 100 calories in the form of ice cream is vastly different from the way it responds to 100 calories in the form of broccoli. The nutrients in these foods determine how they are absorbed and metabolized. For long-term success—and that is what the A-list program is all about—you must care about the long-term metabolic, hormonal, digestive, mental, and overall health aspects of your diet. A calorie is not just a calorie.

3. **Do I need to eat all this food?** *No!* These are your options, but you do not have to force-feed yourself all these foods. Just eat when you are hungry from the lists I have provided. With the A-list Diet, you will hardly even feel hungry.

4. **What about gluten?** The A-List Diet is a program that is naturally gluten free, even in phase three. There are some modifications in the condiment and alcohol section that you would need to make, but otherwise you will be gluten free without any additional effort.

5. **How can I eat out?** Simple! Avoid anything fried or filled with carbohydrates. Ask the server to switch out

the carbohydrate for an extra serving of vegetables and, of course, step away from the bread basket and don't order dessert. Here are examples of foods you can order:

- Italian: Order grilled chicken or fish with grilled vegetables.
- Mexican: Order chicken or beef fajitas—hold the tortillas.
- Pizzeria: Order a salad with chicken, beef, or shrimp.
- Burgers: Ask them to wrap it in lettuce; try turkey or chicken burgers, too.
- Japanese: Order sashimi instead of sushi. Many places can also make rolls without rice.
- Deli: Order a sandwich and throw away the bread (or just order 4 ounces of sliced lunch meat); hard-boiled eggs; tuna salad; chicken salad. Really, there is an endless amount of A-list foods that can be found in a deli.

CHAPTER FIVE

Nutritional Supplements

N utritional supplements are a crucial component of the A-list program. The only ones necessary to ensure success are the protein booster shakes and protein boost shots, which I will discuss in this chapter. But there are lots of others that can help support your progress and help you get even better results.

In order to address the aspects of dieting that are key to being successful, let's break them down into categories:

1. Detox
2. Weight loss
3. Inflammation
4. Alkalization
5. Epigenetics
6. Anti-aging

DETOXIFICATION

Since this is the first step toward weight loss, let me recap what I've already written about in chapter 2. The absolute critical and necessary nutritional supplements for this step of the program are as follows:

1. **DetoxLogic:** You should take two pills three times per day during the first week of the detox and then one pill twice

per day moving forward while you lose weight. As you lose visceral fat, stored toxins will be released into your body. This occurs throughout the weight loss process, not just for the first two weeks. DetoxLogic will help protect your body from those toxins.

2. **Reg'Activ Detox & Liver Health:** This probiotic is the only thing known to science (thus far) that helps your body produce glutathione—a very powerful liver-detoxifying agent. You will need to take one capsule twice per day.

3. **Dr. Ohhira's Probiotics:** There are many probiotics on the market, but this one is truly unique and the only one I recommend to my patients. It has twelve strains of living bacteria that do not need to be refrigerated. Take one capsule twice per day.

4. **MetaMulti Advanced:** This is an amazing multiple vitamin that I created specifically for people with metabolic issues like all of you reading this book. You should be taking two pills three times per day for the entire program, and likely beyond.

Before we move on to the weight-loss supplements, I want you to understand why MetaMulti Advanced is so unique. Most multi-vitamins on the market were designed in the 1940s. When I learned that, I knew we needed a new type of multivitamin to help fight twenty-first-century epidemics like obesity, metabolic syndrome, and type 2 diabetes. It contains optimal doses of the essential nutrients your body needs, supported by science done in this century, not pre–World War II. For instance:

1. **Berberine** works by activating blood sugar–burning enzymes in your bloodstream even when you're at rest.

2. **Cinnamon** enhances the action of berberine by slowing down its absorption. Cinnamon on its own has also been shown to lower blood sugar.

3. **Curcumin** helps support insulin sensitivity and inflammation. I use the patented version known as Meriva, which has demonstrated a fivefold increase in bioavailability in animal trials compared to regular curcumin.

4. **Benfotiamine** helps support the nerve-related discomfort of increased blood sugar (for example, that numbness and tingling you may experience in your fingers and toes).

5. **Purple tea** can help support healthy cholesterol and blood sugar levels. I included a unique, proprietary blend of purple tea known as Alluvia. Alluvia may help you maintain healthy body weight, promote a healthy BMI number, and keep your waistline and hips in check.

6. **GreenSelect®** is a patented green tea extract. A recent study compared two groups of dieters over the course of four weeks. The group dieting and taking GreenSelect® doubled their weight loss compared to the diet-only group.

7. **Niacin** targets both your LDL and HDL cholesterol. According to the Mayo Clinic, niacin not only works to keep your LDL and triglyceride levels healthy but can also help maintain healthy HDL ("good") cholesterol at the same time.

MetaMulti Advanced is also designed to help keep your brain sharp, clear, and focused; maintain a good energy level; keep your joints mobile, limber, and smooth; support eye health; and keep your bones healthy. Overall, it contains thirty-eight specialized vitamins and nutrients designed to combat metabolic syndrome and give you results you can see and feel, all backed up with twenty-first-century science.

WEIGHT LOSS

A variety of nutritional supplements can help support your weight loss efforts. Here are the five "must haves" that I recommend for the A-List Diet:

1. **Protein booster shakes:** Refer to chapter 2 to find the specific shake recipe for your dieting type. One per day is sufficient. This can be taken midday, before or after a workout, or whenever it is convenient for you.

2. **The AM protein boost shot:** Take this every morning, preferably on an empty stomach. If you forget, just take it when you remember, even if you've just eaten. You'll learn more about the AM/PM protein boost shots below.

3. **The PM protein boost shot:** Take this prior to dinner or before going to bed.

4. **BurnLogic:** This is another supplement that I developed for the A-listers, and you should take one tablet twice per day (more on this below).

5. **Robuvit®:** This is an amazing new supplement that I will tell you about shortly. I recommend one tablet per day.

There are other supplements that can certainly aid in the process of weight loss, but these five items are necessary for your success and they are a must for the A-List Diet program. You already know about the protein booster shakes, so let me reveal the powerful protein boost shots, explain the breakthrough ingredients in BurnLogic, and then tell you all about Robuvit®.

Protein Boost Shots

These are the stars of the A-List Diet—the branched-chain amino acids (BCAAs) I've been telling you about. They are the tools that changed my practice and how my patients—and I—manage our weight, and they are going to change your life forever. These protein boost shots are specifically formulated to be taken in the morning and in the evening. They are portable, taste delicious, and, most importantly, are the key to losing weight. These special boost shots that I formulated specifically for my A-listers can be bought online at AListDietBook.com. They are an addition to the protein booster shakes that you can make from ingredients you can buy at ordinary health food stores. There is no other diet program that makes it this simple to lose weight. Yes, food is critical, but these shots take the A-list program to a whole new level of dieting.

Let me share with you what is in them:

THE AM PROTEIN BOOST SHOT
Chocolate

3,500 mg BCAA blend (L-leucine, L-isoleucine, L-valine)
250 mg unsweetened cocoa powder
200 mg dimethylglycine (DMG)

THE PM PROTEIN BOOST SHOT
Pineapple-Mango

3,500 mg BCAA blend (L-leucine, L-isoleucine, L-valine)
250 mg curcumin (95 percent curcuminoids)
200 mg dimethylglycine (DMG)

A Note on the Ingredients

Cocoa—at least in its purest form—is a bona fide health food. Cocoa is a rich source of antioxidant polyphenols and contains almost more antioxidants than any other substance on the planet. Polyphenols identified in cocoa beans and cocoa products comprise mainly catechins, flavonol glycosides, anthocyanins, and procyanidins. This unique flavonoid profile makes it a delicious way to promote healthy high blood pressure, cholesterol, and inflammation, which will keep your heart pumping and maintain healthy blood sugar levels by supporting insulin pathways—all metabolic issues that make cocoa a perfect fit for the A-list morning protein boost shot.

Dimethylglycine (DMG) is an important part of the protein boost shots because it is related to the amino acid glycine. Research shows that it supplies essential methyl groups for modifying, building, and detoxifying the body. DMG also provides these health benefits:

1. Contributes useful building blocks for the biosynthesis of vitamins, hormones, neurotransmitters, antibodies, nucleic acids, and other metabolically active molecules.
2. Supports all aspects of immune response by acting as an antiviral, antibacterial, and anti-fungal agent.
3. Promotes cardiovascular functions by supporting normal triglyceride and cholesterol levels, reducing angina, improving circulation, and decreasing elevated homocysteine levels.
4. Improves oxygenation, thus reducing fatigue and increasing energy for improved physical and mental performance.
5. Supports neurological function and mental clarity by acting as a precursor to the amino acids that are building blocks for neurotransmitters.
6. Acts as an antioxidant against free radicals.
7. Supports detoxification and enhances liver function.

Curcumin is the main spice in curry, one of my favorite foods and something that will keep your weight loss humming along. The only difference between the AM and PM shots (besides the flavor, of course) is the curcumin in the PM shot.

The curcuminoids in turmeric have been shown in study after study to counter many of the factors that contribute to metabolic syndrome. I'm talking about its ability to help reduce belly fat while promoting healthy blood pressure, blood sugar levels, cholesterol, and triglycerides.

Curcumin has strong antioxidant and anti-inflammatory properties, which makes it a key nutrient to help stave off the dangers of metabolic syndrome in several ways: lowering blood sugar, stimulating blood sugar uptake in the cells, stimulating the pancreas to produce insulin, improving how the pancreatic cells function, and reducing insulin resistance.

Having curcumin in your PM shot is a good way to mop up the oxidative stress and help maintain a healthy response to inflammation. This shot will keep your A-list metabolism working until the morning.

Melissa's A-List Diet Story

Melissa, a television and movie star I'm sure you know well since she's constantly on the cover of magazines, had some medical issues. For one, she is perimenopausal, and that makes weight loss quite difficult. While many A-list actors slack off between roles, Melissa can't because perimenopause doesn't allow for that kind of leniency.

Melissa was about to do a role that required her to look fit but one where she needed to be taken seriously—something she might get nominated for. Time for the big guns.

Bottom line: Melissa needed a different protein booster shake than she was taking, and she had fallen into a rut of eating too many acidic foods. I switched her to the shake for the diet challenged and recommended more of the alkalizing foods. Because of perimenopause, she needed to eat more fish, which has more essential fatty acids to help boost metabolism than white meat chicken does, and full-fat dairy. I encouraged her to eat more foods that contain lysine to promote collagen formation, such as nuts, seeds, and eggs, so her skin would look better and to up the ante on the vegetables.

Within two weeks, she looked amazing. She had not only lost the weight necessary for the role, but she didn't need to have a face peel because her skin was radiant. She was thrilled. I was thrilled, too, and the best part is that it was so easy.

BurnLogic

BurnLogic combines the best of the latest "newcomers" to the weight loss scene. Let's take a look at the ingredients:

1. **Green tea extract** contains epigallocatechin gallate (EGCG), an incredibly powerful polyphenol. Green tea contains antioxidants called catechins, which have been shown to significantly decrease BMI, body weight, body fat,

blood pressure, and total cholesterol. In clinical trials, body fat dropped by an impressive 2.36 percent. Other studies showed that green tea can lower insulin concentrations, fasting glucose levels, and long-term blood sugar control.

2. **Green coffee bean extract** contains powerful natural antioxidants. These aren't found in your morning cup of joe; the strongest antioxidant properties are found in an extract from raw, unroasted coffee beans. It's naturally low in caffeine—less than 3 percent—so there's no risk of the caffeine-related jitters. This extract contains more antioxidants than black tea or brewed coffee.

3. **African mango**, otherwise known as *Irvingia gabonensis,* is a fruit from West Africa. It has been used in traditional folk medicine in western Africa for centuries to treat blood sugar disorders. Using fat cells from mice, scientists discovered that an extract from the African mango seeds blocks fat buildup by mediating a receptor that influences fat storage and glucose metabolism. It also balances levels of leptin and adiponectin—two key fat-regulating hormones. *Irvingia gabonensis* restores appropriate hunger signaling and fires up your body's metabolism.

4. **Raspberry ketone** is an aromatic compound that gives raspberries—and other fruits, including blackberries and cranberries—their distinctive smell. Early research done in mice showed that raspberry ketone supplements prevented both weight gain and the accumulation of visceral fat and prevented fat build-up in the liver. Later research revealed its ability to stimulate secretion of the hormone adiponectin—a hormone critical to appetite control and efficient metabolism.

These four ingredients in BurnLogic work on different parts of the fat-burning mechanisms and also the various complexities of weight loss and management. Weight loss is about getting your body to work the way it's supposed to—diet is the cornerstone for that, and then supplements support that.

Robuvit®

Robuvit® is a patented, all-natural extract from French oak trees. Specifically, it comes from oak trees called *Quercus robur*, which are grown sustainably in France's Massif Central forests. These oak trees are standardized to contain at least 20 percent roburins—a type of flavonoid. Researchers think roburins might actually change the function of ribosomes, our bodies' cellular protein factories. Ribosomes help our cells produce energy, and roburins can help overcome one of the most common "side effects" of being overweight: fatigue. The roburins were found to reduce oxidative stress, which is associated with obesity, metabolic syndrome, and cardiovascular disease.

Robuvit® works well for weight loss since it's a detoxifier that supports your liver and lymphatic system, improves your mood, reduces oxidative stress (which makes weight loss easier), and gives you more energy. The reason it can give you more energy is somewhat of a complicated process and is related to the effects roburins have on the powerhouses of our cells (mitochondria). These cells generate energy from food stuffs, especially fats, which keeps muscles, neurons, and all organs operating well.

The urolithins from Robuvit® cause a more efficient method of building new mitochondria so our cells stay more efficient at burning fat and giving us energy. In fact, Robuvit® has been demonstrated to significantly elevate energy for individuals who suffer from chronic fatigue.

A 2014 study conducted on ninety-one people with at least five primary chronic fatigue syndrome symptoms found that six months of supplementation with Robuvit® (200 milligrams a day) had the following significant effects—pay close attention to the last one:

- 18 percent less weakness and exhaustion
- 29 percent reduction in short-term memory impairment
- 51 percent reduction in joint pain
- 33 percent fewer headaches
- 38 percent reduction in dizziness
- 40 percent less weight fluctuation

Of course, right now no one besides me thinks of using it for weight loss. This is another reason why the A-List Diet and its secrets work—I am always on the lookout for the newest innovations in weight loss. And some of them work in what may seem like mysterious ways. But there is always a method to my madness, and that's for all of us to feel and look the best we can.

Other Key Weight Loss Supplements

While there are many we can talk about, I have been practicing nutritional medicine and weight loss for more than twenty years, and I am going to list only the supplements that I have found to be the most effective with my patients:

1. **Macadamia nut oil** is the only oil I use in my kitchen. It has the highest level of healthy monounsaturated fatty acids (MUFAs) of any oil. That's why when my patients start using macadamia nut oil for all their cooking, those stubborn extra pounds seem to melt off—and why it's an ingredient in the daily protein booster shakes. I wrote an entire book about this ingredient (*The Hamptons Diet*), so I won't spend a lot of time discussing it here.

   Macadamia nut oil is much more versatile than olive oil. Its smoke point is about 40 degrees higher on average than olive oil. So you can safely use it for just about any cooking method—searing, browning, sautéing, frying, and baking—without worrying about losing the health benefits. It has a rich, buttery flavor that isn't overpowering, and I use it extensively in the recipe section of this book.

2. **Astaxanthin** has been shown to positively affect metabolic syndrome. It has significant effects on white adipose tissue by decreasing the size of the fat cells. It has also been shown to significantly reduce blood pressure and fasting blood glucose level, and to improve insulin resistance and insulin sensitivity, making it easier to lose weight. Studies also showed an improved adiponectin level, a significant increase in high-density lipoprotein cholesterol, and a significant decrease in triglyceride levels. I recommend 4 milligrams of astaxanthin per day.

3. **Carnitine** helps your body release fat for fuel and powers up your mitochondria, which are your cellular energy hubs. This amino acid is found in red meat and dairy, but I also recommend taking 500 to 1,000 milligrams of L-carnitine in supplement form three times per day, unless it is found in your protein booster shake.

4. **Coenzyme Q10 (CoQ10)** is found in every cell in your body. This powerful antioxidant is vital to your metabolism, and helps your body release stored fat for fuel. CoQ10 likely lowers your risk of coronary artery disease by helping combat oxidative stress that can damage the heart and arteries. Therefore, it is needed for weight loss and weight management.

5. **Glutamine** is my go-to rescue remedy for sugar addicts, and this amino acid is your first line of defense against sugar cravings. It's a world-class craving killer for a few different reasons. For starters, it is able to inhibit insulin release, which prevents hard blood-sugar crashes. These are the same crashes that often trigger intense cravings for sugar. Glutamine also stimulates your body to release stored glucose in order to get low blood sugar back on track. Finally, glutamine is able

to stand in for sugar itself when your body really needs the energy. That's why I recommend glutamine to my dieting patients—500 milligrams three times a day (in addition to what may be in your protein booster shake), and again whenever you get the urge to grab a cookie or candy bar.

INFLAMMATION

Inflammation is a key reason you are overweight or have difficulty with weight management. The A-List Diet is the best way to reduce inflammation. However, there are four inflammation-fighting supplements that I recommend you take every day:

1. **Fish oil** will help you achieve an optimal balance of omega-6 and omega-3 fatty acids, which is one of the most crucial keys to keeping inflammation under control. The Standard American Diet is packed with the former, so you need to make sure you're getting plenty of the latter.

    Fish oil is the best source of the omega-3 fatty acids EPA (eicosapentaenoic acid) and DHA (docosahexaenoic acid) necessary to balance out those pro-inflammatory omega-6s. For fish oil supplements, check the label for the EPA/DHA content—don't go by total fish oil content. You need 3,000 milligrams of EPA/DHA (not just fish oil) per day. A product with a 3:2 ratio of EPA to DHA is ideal. If you are a vegan, the best product I have seen for providing the necessary omega-3s is Dr. Ohhira's Essential Living Oils.

2. **Vitamin D₃** plays a role in pain and inflammation. One study concluded that people with low levels of vitamin D aren't able to regulate inflammation. But people whose levels are within the normal range can keep inflammation from raging out of control, making this an ideal supplement for anyone who wants to lose weight. It has also been shown to help make people happier and therefore less prone to

bouts of "diet fatigue" than they might normally experience. And, if you live in most of the United States, you can get enough vitamin D only in the summer months, and that's if you sunbathe practically naked without sunscreen for twenty minutes every day. There aren't many foods that contain adequate amounts of vitamin D, so supplements are essential. I recommend at least 2,000 to 5,000 IU per day of vitamin D_3. And be sure to get your blood levels checked periodically by your physician. It should be over 50 (I keep my patients in the 80 to 100 range).

3. **Curcumin** has such a powerful disease-fighting punch that it's one of my "desert island" supplements—a list I compile each year of things I could not live without. It is published annually in my monthly newsletter, *Logical Health Alternatives*. Curcumin is so versatile because it is an incredible anti-inflammatory and helps fight oxidative stress. Take it in supplement form (500 milligrams twice per day) if you forget your protein boost shot or aren't taking them. You should cook with it, too—keep a jar of ground turmeric handy. You can toss this versatile spice with roasted vegetables, add it to scrambled eggs, or mix it into chicken soup.

4. **Bromelain** is a pineapple extract best known in the natural medicine world as a digestive enzyme. But it also has powerful anti-inflammatory effects. A dose of 200 milligrams per day is usually plenty.

ALKALIZATION

Getting your body into an alkaline state is a must for the weight loss results you will achieve with the A-List Diet. There are three key supplements to keep you pH balanced. Taking these supplements and eating according to your dieting type will help optimize your body's pH balance, keeping your body in its ideal fat-burning state and maximizing the functioning of all your systems:

1. **Green superfoods** refers to foods like spirulina, chlorella, barley grass, and wheatgrass. These particular greens are your best bet for beating an acidic pH.

   Barlean's Greens is my favorite choice for alkalization. Unlike most other green superfood products, this one was designed specifically for this purpose. I prefer the regular powder (not the chocolate or fruit-flavored varieties), and I recommend 1 tablespoon mixed into water twice per day throughout your A-list experience.

2. **Betaine HCl** is an acid, so I realize this recommendation might seem counterintuitive. But as the main component of gastric acid, HCl helps you digest food properly. Insufficient levels lower your stomach's pH and erode your ability to digest food, absorb nutrients, and fend off harmful bacteria.

   Unfortunately, as we age, we produce less stomach acid. Not only that, but far too many people today are on antacid medications, which make the problem worse. Many of the issues we associate with excess stomach acid—indigestion, heartburn, and so on—are really the byproducts of low HCl. That's why I recommend taking 500 milligrams before each meal. And if you do choose to take it, you must not forget to eat. It should be taken only with full meals, and not snacks.

3. **Deglycyrrhizinated licorice (DGL)** is an extract of licorice root that has been deglycyrrhizinated (it will say that—or DGL—on the label). This simply means that a compound you find in whole licorice, called glycyrrhizin, has been removed. Glycyrrhizin is what gives licorice root its sweetness. And in high doses or with long-term use, it can raise cortisol levels, leading to issues with weight gain, water retention, and high blood pressure.

   DGL, on the other hand, is safe for anyone to take. Typically, it's used to address issues like indigestion, heartburn, and stomach ulcers. These are all signs of gut inflammation and are common in patients with highly acidic diets. The DGL I use is a standardized herbal extract of about 380 milligrams per capsule. I recommend taking one before each meal.

EPIGENETICS

There are two things that can help with the changes in the expression of our DNA that occur when we eat poorly, have too much stress in our lives, or just plain live in this toxic world.

The first I have already mentioned, and that is taking a good multivitamin. The second product that helps keep your telomeres intact is something called astragaloside IV. It is made from astragalus, which you may have heard of as it has been used in traditional Chinese medicine for centuries. Astragaloside IV is the active ingredient that has been shown to be a telomerase activator, and you can get it in a product called Telomere Benefits from DaVinci Labs. Astragaloside IV also supports memory, energy, muscle strength, stamina, recovery and repair, stress management, immune system, and the cardiovascular system.

While these are by far the two most important supplements to support your telomeres, there are others: SAM-e, folate, methionine, vitamin B_{12}, biotin, curcumin, resveratrol, genistein, alpha-GPC, and betaine HCl.

ANTI-AGING

Who doesn't want to look younger? But it is more important to be younger on the inside. That, to me, is the real measure of how well you are aging. Looking good is one thing—feeling good and having your body function the way it is supposed to is another. The main battle with aging well is your diet and your body's ability to handle inflammation and oxidative stress. Since I have already spent quite a bit of time on those two subjects, these last two supplements are for the pros in the group who want to be as healthy as they can be.

CocoaLogic

This is a powder that I formulated to take advantage of all the health benefits of cocoa and combine them with some anti-aging amino acids. I've already told you why cocoa is so good for you, but let me briefly mention some of the science:

1. A high dose of cocoa significantly improved blood vessel function and blood flow after just two hours in one clinical trial.
2. Smelling chocolate was correlated with reduced levels of ghrelin, the body's hunger hormone. In other words, just the scent of chocolate can help curb appetite.
3. People who eat chocolate on a daily basis can reduce the amount of food they eat at meals—and between-meal snacks—according to one neuroscientist.
4. When scientists studied chocolate's effects on mood, they found people in the "high-dose" chocolate group reported feeling calmer and more content.
5. According to a 2011 study, the most powerful form of cocoa contains three times more antioxidant flavonols than any other superfood.
6. A 2013 study in the journal *Neurology* found that cocoa polyflavanols supported cognitive function—in just thirty days.
7. A review published in 2013 of seventy human clinical trials spanning twelve years found that cocoa helps arteries stay healthy and blood pressure steady, and may even help keep cholesterol levels in check.

The anti-aging amino acids in CocoaLogic play a direct role in every process related to aging: energy, skin health, metabolism, memory. Let's take a look at each one:

1. **Glutamine** is the most abundant amino acid in the body. When you're young and healthy, your body makes plenty of glutamine. But as you age and during times of extreme stress (like injury, critical illness, or surgery) you need even more glutamine. This amino acid can also slow down the aging process of the skin—which means fewer wrinkles and less hair loss—and support mood by helping your brain produce the anxiety-soothing neurotransmitter gamma-aminobutyric acid (GABA). Research shows that glutamine supplementation can raise your human growth hormone (HGH) levels significantly.

2. **Arginine** has a slightly different but equally crucial role in the anti-aging game. For starters, it's necessary for the production of creatine, an essential energy source for muscles. Arginine plays a critical part in the release of nitric oxide (NO), and NO is a requirement for proper functioning of the endothelium (the technical term for the cells that line your blood vessels). In other words, arginine is essential for healthy circulation. And when your body gets a steady flow of blood and oxygen, you feel vibrant and energized. Together, arginine and nitric oxide play an integral role in a strong immune system, improved insulin sensitivity, a sharp memory and clear mind, strong hair growth, energy and stamina, stronger libido, better sperm motility, and vaginal lubrication.

3. **Ornithine** converts into arginine in your body. In tandem, these two amino acids play a crucial role in liver detoxification. More specifically, this combination helps convert harmful ammonia—a natural byproduct of protein breakdown—into urea in order to clear it from the blood. Ornithine on its own can also boost sexual potency and arousal in men, not to mention improve sleep and help with wound healing.

4. **Glycine** is a key component of collagen. Without enough glycine, damaged tissue isn't rejuvenated, which means your skin starts to sag and wrinkle. Glycine also plays an important part in brain health and cognitive ability. Glycine converts into dimethylglycine (DMG), which, as I mentioned earlier, plays an important role in healthy hormone balance.

5. **Lysine** boosts collagen production, which helps keep skin taut and firm, and increases calcium uptake. In effect, this amino acid energizes your body's bone-building cells— remember, bone is made of collagen, too—especially in combination with arginine. And both men and women need strong bones.

As for the doses, this is what you need on a daily basis to achieve the desired effect:

- 6,000 mg L-glutamine
- 1,000 mg L-arginine
- 1,000 mg L-ornithine
- 1,250 mg L-lysine
- 1,000 mg L-glycine

CocoaLogic combines all five of these anti-aging amino acids— the very building blocks of life itself—along with one of the world's strongest superfoods, premium dark cocoa powder, in one delicious place and in those exact doses. My patients love this combination, and it's a great addition to the A-list protocol. Once scoop per day will set you on the path to youth.

Pycnogenol®

If you are a fan of mine, you know I am a very big proponent of this nutritional supplement. Pycnogenol® is a very powerful super-antioxidant made from an extract of the bark of the French maritime pine tree. It works on the collagen and elastin throughout the body, making it the perfect anti-aging supplement. You see, collagen and elastin are in every part of our body, from our skin (which is why we get wrinkles as we age, thanks to the breakdown of collagen and elastin) to our blood vessels and capillaries.

This supplement can help support brain health and blood vessel health, ease menopause symptoms, manage blood sugar levels, boost heart health, improve skin tone, fight colds and flu, and even help with jet lag. And that's just to name a few of its many benefits—there are over 250 clinical trials to support what Pycnogenol® does. It has always made my list of desert island supplements, and you should be taking 100 milligrams per day.

SLEEP

Getting a good night's rest is part of the A-list program. Sleep is one of the most critical—and most overlooked—parts of losing weight (and of good health in general). And bad sleep habits can wreak havoc on your efforts to slim down.

Sadly, according to the National Institutes of Health, almost half of adults age sixty and older have difficulty falling or staying asleep. Obviously, you need quality zzz's to feel vibrant, energized, and youthful. But getting enough sleep is also critical for preserving a young-looking, luminous complexion. Your body's collagen production actually depends on a complex series of events that take place while you sleep. So sleep is truly one of the most effective ways to combat wrinkles.

We've discussed epigenetics, and getting enough sleep is a perfect example of how you can help overcome an inherited genetic tendency to gain weight. Here's what researchers have found:

- Those who slept less increased their genetic risk of higher BMI.
- Those who slept longer had a lower BMI than those who slept less.

- More than nine hours of sleep resulted in the least weight gain.
- Seven to nine hours of sleep reduced weight gain in 40 percent of the participants.
- 70 percent of those who got less than seven hours of sleep gained weight.

However, be careful that you're not sleeping in late, which has also been linked to gaining weight, in order to get those extra zzz's. Early to bed and early to rise is a good adage to follow for health and wellness, and just by following the A-list program, you will sleep better. Better quality of food and decreased inflammation will help account for that. But for those nights when it is not going to happen, there are a number of safe, natural supplements that can help you get good, quality sleep:

1. **5-HTP** is an amino acid (see, they are everywhere and affect everything!) that is found in milk and turkey. It has been shown to work on the neurotransmitters in the brain to help you get a good rest. Start by taking 100 milligrams at bedtime and increase by 100 milligrams a day until you see the effects; most people don't need more than 1,000 milligrams, but you can safely go as high as 5,000 milligrams.
2. **SAM-e** is another amino acid that works on neurotransmitter levels to regulate cortisol so that the biorhythm of your cortisol synchronizes correctly, allowing you to fall asleep at the appropriate time. Take 400 milligrams every morning.
3. **ETAS** is a novel enzyme-processed asparagus stem extract that may help us sleep by reducing stress. In clinical trials, this new supplement improved sleep onset, early awakening, sleep time, and sleep quality, and decreased distress caused

by insomnia and interference with daily functioning. Take 200 milligrams before bedtime.

4. **Theanine** is another amino acid and is the calming agent found in green tea. Take 200 milligrams in the morning and another 200 milligrams thirty minutes before bed.

5. **Melatonin** is generated by your body not just to help you sleep but also to aid the immune system. Unfortunately, production takes a nosedive as you age. I recommend starting with 3 milligrams at bedtime and working your way up, if needed, to a maximum of 21 milligrams. And if this doesn't help, there are time-released versions that seem to work better in some people.

While I can go on and on, the one thing that should be clear is that in order to take control of your weight loss, weight management, and overall health, a combination of diet and nutritional supplements can't be beat—especially doing it in A-list style.

SUPPLEMENT SUMMARY

Phase One: Detoxification (week one)

1. DetoxLogic (or something similar): two pills three times per day
2. Reg'Activ Detox & Liver Health: one capsule twice per day
3. Dr. Ohhira's Probiotics: one capsule twice per day
4. MetaMulti Advanced (or something similar): two tablets three times per day

Phase Two: Weight Loss (week two and beyond)

1. AM protein boost shot: one per day
2. PM protein boost shot: one per day
3. Protein booster shake for your dieting type: one per day

4. BurnLogic: one tablet twice per day
5. Robuvit®: one tablet per day
6. DetoxLogic: one pill three times per day for the first week, then one pill twice per day
7. Reg'Activ Detox & Liver Health: one capsule twice per day
8. Dr. Ohhira's Probiotics: one capsule twice per day
9. MetaMulti Advanced: two tablets three times per day
10. Fish oil: 1,500 milligrams of EPA/DHA twice per day
11. Vitamin D_3: 2,000 to 5,000 IU per day
12. Barlean's Greens: one serving twice per day (you can add it to your protein booster shake)
13. CocoaLogic: one scoop per day (you can also add this to your protein booster shake)

The other supplements mentioned in this chapter are very important and can make your weight loss and weight management experience smoother. But I understand they are costly and may be tedious to remember. So, if you can do only a few, choose from this list and never forget the protein boost shots and shakes.

CHAPTER SIX

Tips for Healthier Eating

A s you will recall, the entire basis of the A-List Diet program is having all the amino acids you need and in the right proportions in order to achieve terrific and everlasting results. This is the main difference between the A-List Diet and all the other high-protein diets. Those other diets simply don't take into account the micronutrient breakdown of the foods we eat—and that is the key to long-term success.

While the protein boost shots and the protein booster shakes will provide this necessary balance, it is important that you understand that pretty much everything you eat contains amino acids. They are the building blocks of life, and having the proper balance of amino acids is very important. I understand that not everyone likes to take a lot of nutritional supplement pills, capsules, and powders so, in this chapter, I will provide lists of foods that contain the different amino acids and summarize what they do for you, so you can choose what *you* like to eat.

You can follow my meal plans and recipes—which are full of the essential amino acids and which can be found at the end of the book—or you can use these lists to do it for yourself. Feel free to make substitutions in case you don't like my suggestions or need something different. I have provided you with a good start, but your weight loss journey might take more than just the thirty days I outlined. To make healthy eating choices for life, simply choose from the recommended foods in chapter 4 (if you're trying to lose weight) or chapter 9 (if you're on maintenance). This chapter contains information that will make it even easier for you to achieve your amino acid and weight loss goals.

ESSENTIAL AMINO ACIDS

1. **Phenylalanine** acts as an appetite suppressant by causing the release of an intestinal hormone called cholecystokinin that signals the brain to feel satiated after eating. Phenylalanine should not be taken by pregnant women or those who suffer from high blood pressure, phenylketonuria, melanoma, or anxiety attacks. It should not be eaten if you're taking MAO inhibitor drugs, prescribed for depression. Phenylalanine is found in a variety of foods, including these:

almonds	cheese	peanuts
apples	corn	pineapples
avocados	eggs	pumpkin seeds
bananas	fish	sesame seeds
beets	lima beans	soy products
brown rice	nutritional yeast	spinach
carrots	parsley	tomatoes

2. **Valine** appears to promote glycogen synthesis in muscle cells and has been noted to increase insulin secretion from the pancreas. It plays a role in regulating absorption of other amino acids. Valine helps remove potentially toxic excess nitrogen from the liver and transports it to other tissues in the body as needed. It also stimulates the nervous system and is necessary for proper mental functioning. Foods high in valine include these:

almonds	dandelion greens	parsnips
apples	fish	pomegranates
beans	lamb	pork
beef	lettuce	seeds
beets	mushrooms	soybeans
carrots	nutritional yeast	squash
celery	nuts	tomatoes
cheese	okra	turnips
chicken	parsley	whole grains

3. **Threonine** aids in the creation of collagen and elastin and the production of digestive enzymes. High-threonine foods include these:

alfalfa sprouts	green leafy vegetables	nori
beans	kale	nuts
carrots	lean beef	papayas
celery	lentils	pork
cheese	lettuce (especially iceberg)	seeds
chicken	lima beans	shellfish
collards	liver	soy

4. **Tryptophan** is needed for general growth and development, the production of niacin, and serotonin in the body. High-tryptophan foods include these:

alfalfa sprouts	dandelion greens	oats
beans	eggs	red meat
Brussels sprouts	endive	seeds
carrots	fennel	snap beans
celery	fish	spinach
cheese	lentils	tofu
chicken	nutritional yeast	turkey
chives	nuts	turnips

5. **Methionine** helps form cartilage and may also help prevent hair loss and strengthen nails. A deficiency of methionine can lead to inflammation of the liver, anemia, and graying hair. High-methionine foods include these:

apples	dairy	nuts
beans	eggs	pineapples
beef	filberts	pork
Brazil nuts	fish	shellfish
Brussels sprouts	garlic	sorrel
cabbage	horseradish	soy
cauliflower	kale	turkey
cheese	lamb	watercress
chives		

6. **Leucine** is used in the liver, fat tissue, and muscle tissue. It helps burn visceral fat, which is located in the deepest layers of the body and is the least responsive to dieting and exercise. It also aids in insulin regulation. Leucine promotes the healing of bones, skin, and muscle tissue after traumatic injury, and is often recommended for those recovering from surgery. High-leucine foods include these:

avocados	coconut	pork
beans	fish	seafood
beef	nuts	seeds
cheese	olives	soybeans
chicken	papayas	

7. **Isoleucine** is best known for its ability to increase endurance, help heal and repair muscle tissue, and encourage clotting at the site of injury. It also keeps energy levels stable by helping regulate blood sugar. A deficiency of isoleucine produces symptoms similar to those of hypoglycemia and may include headaches, dizziness, fatigue, depression, confusion, and irritability. Isoleucine is found in these foods:

alfalfa sprouts	fish	seaweed
avocados	game meats	spinach
cheese	lamb	sunflower seeds
chicken	olives	Swiss chard
coconut	pak choi	turkey
crustaceans	papayas	watercress
eggs	pheasant	

8. **Lysine** is involved in the creation of collagen and absorption of calcium. Lysine may also help alleviate herpes simplex infections. Foods high in lysine include these:

alfalfa sprouts	dandelion greens	pears
apples	eggs	pork
apricots	fish	seeds
beans	grapes	shellfish
beets	lean beef	shrimp
carrots	lentils	soy
celery	nuts	spinach
cheese	papayas	turkey
chicken	parsley	turnip greens
cucumber		

9. **Histidine** is used to develop and maintain the myelin sheaths that coat nerve cells and ensure the transmission of messages from the brain to various parts of the body. It is also known to help support proper blood pressure. This amino can be found in these foods:

alfalfa sprouts	chicken	pomegranates
apples	cucumbers	pork
beef	dandelion greens	radishes
beets	endive	spinach
bison	fish	turkey
carrots	garlic	turnip greens
celery	lamb	

CONDITIONAL ESSENTIAL AMINO ACIDS

1. **Arginine** can accelerate insulin secretion, stimulate protein regeneration, and promote the transport of amino acids into the cells. It helps increase the oxygen and blood flow by boosting nitric oxide production, promoting collagen formation, and reducing inflammation, thereby supporting a lower blood pressure. Arginine can be found in these foods:

alfalfa sprouts	dairy	peanuts
beets	green vegetables	pork loin
carrots	leeks	potatoes
celery	lentils	pumpkin seeds
chicken breast	lettuce	radishes
chickpeas	nutritional yeast	soybeans
cucumbers	parsnips	turkey

2. **Cysteine** helps create antioxidants in the body, aids in lowering blood sugar, and can support a lower blood pressure. Cysteine is required to synthesize glutathione, our bodies' major antioxidant, which plays a key role in pretty much everything. High cysteine foods include these:

beef	fish	oats
cheese	kamut	pork
chicken	lamb	soybeans
eggs	legumes	sunflower seeds

3. **Glycine** helps regulate and support blood pressure and is important for the construction of healthy DNA and RNA strands. Glycine is one of the three amino acids that form creatine, which can help promote muscle growth and energy production during exercise. Glycine is also the primary component of collagen, the tissue that makes up most of your skin, tendons, and ligaments. Glycine can help your

body regulate blood sugar levels by controlling the amount of blood sugar that is released into your blood stream from your liver and fat stores. It also provides glucose to skeletal muscle so it can be used for energy. Glycine may benefit people suffering from hypoglycemia (low blood sugar), anemia, and chronic fatigue. Glycine also assists in the production of bile, which helps to digest dietary fatty acids. It is more commonly found in these foods:

beef	mollusks	sesame seeds
chicken	ostrich	spinach
lamb	pork	watercress

4. **Glutamine** functions as a fuel source for fibroblasts and epithelial cells needed for healing. Glutamine helps improve gastrointestinal health because it is a vital nutrient for the intestines to rebuild and repair. It helps heal ulcers and leaky gut, acts as a neurotransmitter in the brain, and helps with memory, focus, and concentration. Glutamine improves irritable bowel syndrome and diarrhea by balancing mucus production. It has been shown to promote muscle growth and decrease muscle wasting, improve athletic performance and recovery from endurance exercise, improve metabolism and cellular detoxification, curb cravings for sugar and alcohol, fight cancer, and improve diabetes and blood sugar. The foods with the most glutamine are these:

asparagus	cottage cheese	turkey
bone broth	grass-fed beef	venison
broccoli rabe	spirulina	wild-caught fish
Chinese cabbage		

5. **Proline** aids the body in breaking down proteins for use in healthy cells. Proline is a precursor for hydroxyproline. The body uses hydroxyproline to make collagen, tendons, and ligaments. Collagen, which contains approximately 15

percent proline, is a key component in our skin, and our skin is the first line of defense against infection. It can also improve skin texture and spur new cell formation. Proline plays an important role in combating arteriosclerosis by enabling arterial cell walls to release fat buildup into the bloodstream, decreasing the size of the blockages to the heart and surrounding vessels. Because collagen is found in the lining of our blood vessels, it helps support a healthy blood pressure. Proline is most commonly found in these foods:

asparagus	cheese	lamb
beef	chicken	pork
broccoli rabe	chives	watercress
cabbage	gelatin	

6. **Tyrosine** is an amino acid that is used to produce noradrenaline and dopamine—two important neurotransmitters. Some studies suggest that extra tyrosine may help improve people's memory under stress. High-tyrosine foods include these:

beans	fish	seeds
beef	kidney beans	soybeans
cheese	lamb	spinach
chicken	mustard greens	turnip greens
dairy	nuts	watercress
eggs	pork	whole grains

OTHER AMINO ACIDS

1. **Alanine** is mostly synthesized by muscle cells from lactic acid. It is considered the most important nutrient for amino acid metabolism in the blood, together with L-glutamine. Once synthesized, alanine is absorbed via the liver and converted to pyruvate, which is critical for the production

of glucose and blood sugar management. It has also been shown to enhance athletic performance by boosting carnosine levels, which helps reduce fatigue. Alanine is most abundantly found in these foods:

beef	poultry	wheat germ
fish	soy	white mushrooms
parsley	sunflower seeds	

2. **Aspartic acid** is thought to help promote metabolism and is sometimes used to treat fatigue and depression. Aspartic acid plays an important role in the Krebs cycle, during which other amino acids and biochemicals—such as asparagine, arginine, lysine, methionine, threonine, and isoleucine—are synthesized. Aspartic acid moves the coenzyme nicotinamide adenine dinucleotide (NADH) molecules from the main body of the cell to the mitochondria, where it is used to generate adenosine triphosphate (ATP), the fuel that powers all cellular activity. This amino acid helps transport minerals needed to form healthy RNA and DNA to the cells, and strengthens the immune system by promoting increased production of immunoglobulins and antibodies. Aspartic acid keeps your mind sharp by increasing concentrations of NADH in the brain, which is thought to boost the production of neurotransmitters and chemicals needed for normal mental functioning. It also removes excess toxins from the cells, particularly ammonia, which is very damaging to the brain and nervous system. This amazing amino can be found in these foods:

asparagus	halibut	spinach
bamboo shoots	lentils	swamp cabbage
cod	mung beans	tilapia
crab	orange roughy	tuna
egg whites	peppers	whitefish

3. **Asparagine** helps maintain balance or equilibrium. It is also essential for the proper functioning and health of our nerves and is essential to the synthesis of a large number of other proteins. It is found in these foods:

asparagus	legumes	red meat
dairy	nuts	soy
eggs	potatoes	whole grains
fish	poultry	

4. **Glutamic acid** helps support a lower blood pressure and contributes to the health of the immune and digestive systems, as well as energy production. It's the most common neurotransmitter found within the spinal cord and brain. Glutamic acid is also important in the synthesis of gamma-aminobutyric acid (GABA), which is a natural calming agent. This amino can be found in these foods:

avocados	kelp	salmon
beans	lentils	sirloin
chicken breast	lobster	sunflower seeds
dairy products	meat	turkey breast
eggs	peanuts	wakame
fish	poultry	walnuts

5. **Serine** is especially important to proper functioning of the brain and central nervous system. Serine helps form the phospholipids needed to make every cell in your body. The proteins used to form the brain, as well as the protective myelin sheaths that cover the nerves, contain serine. Serine is also needed to produce tryptophan, an amino acid that is used to make serotonin, our happy brain chemical. Both serotonin and tryptophan shortages have been linked to depression, insomnia, confusion, and anxiety. It is also involved in the function of RNA and DNA, fat and fatty

acid metabolism, muscle formation, and the maintenance of a healthy immune system. Research suggests that low levels of serine may contribute to chronic fatigue syndrome and fibromyalgia. Serine helps produce immunoglobulins and antibodies for a strong immune system, and also aids in the absorption of creatine, a substance made from amino acids that helps build and maintain all the muscles in the body, including the heart. Serine can be found in these foods:

baby squash	cuttlefish	quail
bamboo shoots	egg whites	seaweed
buffalo	elk	turkey breast
cottage cheese	kidney beans	watercress
cream cheese	pike	

THE IMPORTANCE OF PROTEIN

As you can see, we can get amino acids from both animal and vegetable sources of foods—even fruits. The A-list program ensures that you get enough protein in your diet, but you get the right kind. Bear in mind that the recommended daily allowance (RDA) for every macro- and micronutrient was established in the 1940s during World War II when we were concerned with what Americans minimally needed in times of rationing in order to be healthy. These RDAs simply have no relevance to our current lifestyle. So don't be alarmed to find you may be eating a lot more than the RDA of protein.

Protein is such a huge part of the zeitgeist that we are even starting to look at the health benefits of eating insect proteins such as crickets. Protein is here to stay, although it wasn't too long ago that health experts were fearful of protein. You need look no further back than the 1980s when animal protein was considered deadly. Science has evolved so quickly, and the A-List Diet takes advantage of all the latest protein and amino acid science.

When you vary your proteins—between grass-fed lean beef, pasture-raised chicken breast, line-caught tuna, wild salmon, pastured pork, for example—you vary your micronutrients and your amino acids and crank up your metabolism, leading to leaner muscle and shedding of visceral fat.

There is evidence to suggest that 0.7 to 1 gram of protein per pound of body weight is ideal for most of us each day, more if you are trying to bulk up. Ideally, your protein intake should be divided into four feedings, with less at breakfast and lunch and more at dinner. The fourth dose of protein can come in the form of a snack after the gym.

THE ALKALINE WAY

To further enhance your new way of eating, I ask that you choose more food from the alkaline categories than the acidic ones. Here's the A-List Diet's alkaline cheat sheet. Of course, if you follow the meal plans I've outlined and take the nutritional supplements, you will be well balanced in this respect and can use this chart simply as a reference for grocery shopping or eating out.

Eat More	Eat Less
aged cheese, butter, cream, goat cheese	cottage cheese, ice cream, new cheese, processed cheese
arugula, asparagus, beets, bell peppers, broccoli, Brussels sprouts, burdock, cabbage, cauliflower, celery, chives, cilantro, collard greens, cucumbers, daikon, eggplant, endive, garlic, ginger, jicama, kale, kohlrabi, lettuce, mushrooms, mustard greens, onions, parsley, parsnip, radishes, rutabagas, scallions, seaweed and other sea vegetables, squash, sweet potatoes, taro root, turmeric, turnips, yams	carrots, chard, lima beans, peanuts, rhubarb, snow peas, spinach, zucchini
apples, apricots, avocados, blackberries, blueberries, boysenberries, cantaloupe, cherries, grapes, grapefruit, honeydew, lemons, limes, mangoes, nectarines, olives, oranges, peaches, pears, persimmons, raspberries, raw tomatoes, strawberries, tangerines, watermelon	canned fruit, cooked tomato, cranberries, dates, dried fruit, figs, guava, plums, pomegranates, prunes
amaranth, brown rice, buckwheat, kamut, kasha, millet, oat, quinoa, sago, spelt, wheat	all-purpose flour, barley, barley groats, bleached flour, corn, rye, maize, oat bran
boar, chicken eggs, elk, fish, game, gelatin, goose, lamb, mollusks, organ meat, shellfish, turkey, venison, wild duck	beef, chicken, lobster, mussels, pheasant, pork, squid, veal
lentils, mung beans	adzuki beans, black-eyed peas, fava beans, green peas, kidney beans, navy beans, pinto beans, chickpeas, lima beans, white beans, red beans, soybeans
almond oil, avocado oil, borage oil, clarified butter, coconut oil, cod liver oil, flaxseed oil, macadamia nut oil, olive oil, evening primrose oil	Brazil nut oil, chestnut oil, cottonseed oil, palm oil, soy oil, superheated vegetable oils (especially canola)
almonds, cashews, chestnuts, poppy seeds, pumpkin seeds, sesame seeds	Brazil nuts, hazelnuts, peanuts, pecans, pine nuts

INFLAMMATION FIGHTING

If you ever hope to lose weight and maintain that weight loss, reducing inflammation is critical. You can start slashing inflammation right at the supermarket by cutting out the processed, packaged foods. Instead, focus on whole, natural, minimally processed foods. This one simple step alone will make a huge difference in easing inflammation throughout your body.

And it's not as difficult as it might seem to make the switch. You've probably heard this advice before, but shopping the "perimeter" of the grocery store is the simplest way to bypass most processed foods altogether. Avoid "foods" like crackers, granola bars, cereals, bottled salad dressings, and so on—all the products that fill up the center aisles in the supermarket. Stock your shopping cart with vegetables, fruit, cheese, meat, and seafood.

SOME EPIGENETIC FOOD CHOICES

You should try to eat as many foods as you can that have these potent phytochemicals in them to help with your genetic makeup:

1. **Folate** can be found in leafy greens, green tea, brightly colored vegetables like asparagus and spinach, and strawberries.
2. **Methionine** (another important amino acid) can be found in eggs, halibut, chicken, turkey, tuna, and freshwater fish such as pike.
3. **Vitamin B$_{12}$** can be found in eggs, beef, salmon, tuna, cod, lamb, shellfish, and sardines.
4. **Choline** can be found in eggs, shrimp, scallops, chicken, turkey, cod, tuna, salmon, beef, leafy greens, green tea, collard greens, and Brussels sprouts.
5. **Resveratrol** can be found in red fruits such as grapes and blueberries, peanuts, spices, and dark cocoa.

6. **Sulforaphane** is a very important cancer fighter, and most people's favorite source is broccoli. But it can also be found in other leafy greens such as kale and kohlrabi, as well as in green tea and horseradish.
7. **Isothiocyanate** can be found in horseradish, mustard, radishes, Brussels sprouts, watercress, and capers.
8. **Genistein** can be found in legumes such as peanuts and soybeans.

THE TRUTH BEHIND ORGANIC

Is buying organic worth it? This is a tricky question. The federal standards are actually quite lax, and why wouldn't you expect that from our government? According to federal guidelines, an organic product can have nonorganic ingredients.

Caveat Emptor

The U.S. Department of Agriculture (USDA—one of my least favorite governmental agencies) recently "clarified" (by which I mean "loosened") the definition of organic. It has decided that it is okay to have antibiotics in dairy cows, certain chemicals in pesticides, and nonorganic fish meal in livestock feed. Fish meal can contain preservatives, PCBs, and mercury. This basically means that what your animals are eating doesn't have to be organic, but the end product can still be called organic. Makes no sense, right? Unless you are a government official, I suppose.

These subtle changes to the standards also allow organic dairy animals to be treated for disease with any drug, including antibiotics and growth hormones, and remain on the organic farm as long as the producer waits twelve months to sell their milk.

The industry argues that they could lose up to 40 percent of their calves unless they are allowed to use drugs. They say it is more humane. However, what should really happen is that if the cow gets sick, it should be treated and made to leave the herd—which is what Horizon Organic does. And you simply don't know which farms are sticking with the standards and which aren't, unless you are willing to do a lot of research.

Let's talk about the ridiculousness of what they are allowing with pesticides in relationship to organic. There are four classes of pesticides:

1. Contains ingredients known to be toxic
2. Contains ingredients with a high probability of toxicity
3. Contains ingredients of unknown toxicity
4. Contains ingredients that cause little or no harm

Previously, only category 4 was allowed on organic farms. Now, the second and third categories are allowed. And here's a twist you may find fascinating: The manufacturers are not required to list the inert ingredients on their food labels. Only they and the Environmental Protection Agency (EPA) know, and the EPA is not permitted to let us know. How does that make any sense? The EPA and a chemical company know what goes into our foods, but we don't. Whose side do you think the government is on? Certainly not ours when it comes to helping us eat healthier.

Despite what I just told you, organic foods are inherently more nutritious. In fact, brand-new research shows that organic crops and foods contain up to 69 percent more antioxidants than conventional crops grown with pesticides. So we're talking about nearly 70 percent more disease-fighting power. A team of UK researchers found that the antioxidant boost you get from switching to organic products could be the equivalent of eating one or two extra servings of fruit and veggies every day. You could also significantly reduce your exposure to nitrates, nitrites, and toxic heavy metals—like lead, mercury, and cadmium—by eating organic crops.

Local versus Organic

These two terms aren't interchangeable, and they mean two totally different things. "Local" means nothing other than that the food was grown or produced near you. It doesn't necessarily mean that it's organic and/or pesticide-free.

And on the flip side of this coin, "organic" doesn't always indicate that the food is locally sourced. In fact, a lot of organic produce on store shelves comes from California or Mexico. While California may be local to some of you, it isn't local to me.

Because of this confusion and willy-nilly federal standards, I recommend buying locally sourced food. In fact, I often choose non-organic local food over organic food that travels a long distance to my plate. Fresh, local food is packed with live enzymes you won't find in food that has spent weeks in crates being shipped across the globe.

There's simply no substitute for knowing where your food is coming from. So, I've found a local farm where I get my produce and meat. That way, I know where my food is coming from and exactly how the animals are treated and how the fruits and vegetables are grown. It may sound extreme, but it's not as difficult as it might sound. And besides farmers' markets, there are many local food cooperatives that focus on local and seasonal crops that will even deliver directly to your door. Community-supported agriculture (CSA) groups are everywhere, and many are even year round, with hydroponic produce in some cases to augment the harvests. In the Resources section, I list a great website that you can use to find a CSA near you. Wherever you decide to get your food, don't be afraid to ask tough questions.

Next time you're at a local farmers' market or farm stand, here are three questions to ask before you buy. You can also ask these questions about specific products you find in natural food stores and supermarkets. They may or may not have the information readily available. If there's any doubt, wait and contact the manufacturer/producer directly.

1. Do you use growth hormones, antibiotics, pesticides, or herbicides in the production of the food you sell?

2. Is the beef you sell grass-fed *and* grass-finished? Antibiotic- and hormone-free meat is generally clearly labeled as such. But things get murky when you start talking about grass versus grain feeding. Unfortunately, many farmers advertise their cows as grass-fed even if they're "finished" on grain. (In other words, these cows grazed for most of their lives but were transitioned to grain feeding before slaughter to fatten them up.) But grain finishing does impact the quality of the beef—and not for the better, either. So if you want a truly healthy product, you want beef from cows that are fed and finished on grass, which means they eat nothing but grass their entire lives up until the day they are slaughtered. That is a cut of meat worth paying more for and a true health food.

3. Are the eggs/chicken you sell pasture raised? Chickens are not vegetarians. They like to peck and forage, and bugs are a big part of their natural diet. It means nothing if they're raised outside of cages if their feed is vegetarian. For optimal nutrition, they must be "pastured," which means they're free to roam and forage on the farm.

Affordability

The price gap between unhealthy, packaged, processed foods and fresh, organic, healthier options has grown much wider over the last ten years. While healthy foods have always been more expensive than their unhealthier counterparts, the size of the price gap between the two has increased by a whopping 28.6 percent in the past ten years. This gap isn't just unacceptable—it's an outrage.

Unfortunately, the price disparity between junk food and whole, natural food in the United States shouldn't surprise anyone. After all, our government subsidizes the primary ingredients in processed foods—wheat, corn, sugar, soybeans, and rice—to the tune of billions of dollars per year. Not only are these the most genetically modified foods, they're also the ones that research has directly linked to a laundry list of illnesses (and to six of the top ten leading causes of death in the United States). Organic farming must be subsidized. There has to be a more efficient, cost-effective way of getting organic, healthier foods from the farm to the table or we will always have the "trendiness" price differential.

The high prices for healthy and nutritious food are a serious cause of the obesity epidemic. A report out of the UK compared retail food prices dating back as far as thirty years and found similar trends in the UK, United States, Brazil, China, Mexico, and Korea. And, not surprisingly, the healthy stuff is going up in price, while the unhealthy food is getting cheaper by the minute. On a global scale, the cost of some processed foods has dropped by up to 20 percent. Compare that to a 91 percent rise in vegetable prices in Brazil, China, Korea, and Mexico. And here's another alarming side-by-side stat: The price of vegetables has risen by a whopping 199 percent in the past thirty years, while the cost of ice cream has fallen by 50 percent. With statistics like that, it's hard to really blame people for the obesity epidemic.

However, I would like to point this out: We are a nation that prides itself on cheap food. Right after World War II, we spent almost 40 percent of our income on food—now it's less than 10 percent. And we have never been fatter or unhealthier. At some point, you have to decide: Do you want that new gadget or do you want to be healthy?

I know organic fruits and vegetables can be expensive. But I do need to reiterate something I've noted before: If you can't afford organic fruits and vegetables, don't give up and dive backward into a bin of powdered donuts. Buy nonorganic fruits and vegetables instead. It's not as good as organic, but it's way better than eating no fruits and veggies at all. If you're still spending a little more on good food even after buying nonorganic, remember this: You're likely saving on future doctor bills.

As for the A-list program, you can use whatever food you can afford. Just know that the better the ingredients, the better the taste and the better the health outcome. The weight loss will occur no matter what. As a doctor, I can't help but want you to be the best you can be.

CHAPTER SEVEN

Food Truths

FOOD CONFUSION

Who isn't confused about food? One day a certain food is good for you and the next day that food will kill you. I call it the demonization and deification effect that we like to do in America with pretty much anything. We find it impossible to live in a world that is gray. We like things black and white. But nutritional science isn't black and white. Medicine isn't black and white. When you consider the number of people on the planet, it is foolish to think that we can all be on the same diet. That's why even the A-list program outlines six separate diet types.

PROTEIN

All your protein should come from animal protein sources, preferably leaner animal proteins. That's not to say that you can't throw in the occasional plant-based protein, but animal proteins contain all the essential amino acids that you need to burn fat. It's going to be hard to talk protein without talking about fat, but we will leave fat until the next section.

The amino acids in protein are the building blocks of muscle. Muscle is good for fat burning because it routinely takes away energy from fat cells to work. It specifically does this from belly fat cells in order to keep it pumped up. Your belly fat hates muscle because muscle stores energy in the form of glycogen that your belly fat would love to turn into more fat cells.

When you eat protein, you are burning a lot of calories. Digesting protein uses 25 percent of the protein calories you just consumed. Carbohydrates, on the other hand, use about 10 percent of their calories to metabolize themselves. The ability to burn more calories even at rest is a no-brainer way of eating for me.

Protein keeps you fuller longer. Studies show that those who eat higher-protein breakfasts or those who eat higher-protein snacks in the afternoon have more energy, are less hungry afterward, and can generally wait longer for their next meal. It's hard to get a more concentrated form of vitamins and minerals than from animal protein that's been fed well. Clearly, anything consumed in excess can make us sick, and meat is no exception. And I'm sure you've heard about studies claiming that eating meat at every meal increases your risk of diabetes, heart disease, obesity, and cancer. But the truth is, it is not the animal protein that is the problem; it is how that animal has been fed.

Beef/Pork/Lamb

The typical cow is fed corn rather than the grass it was meant to eat to fatten her up. So, let's ask ourselves: If the cow is fed grain and corn to fatten it up, doesn't it make sense that you will fatten up, too, if you eat that way?

Corn-fed animal meat is very high in pro-inflammatory omega-6 fatty acids, which increase fatty liver and stowaway sugar. The marbling that is so prized in steakhouses is muscle insulin resistance. Or metabolic syndrome. If you want metabolic syndrome, just eat food from animals with the same issue. Red meat isn't bad for you—the way the cow is treated creates meat that is unhealthy.

Chicken/Other Fowl

I don't want to generalize to all fowl since there may be some that are fed well. Sadly, though, the majority of commercially raised chickens, turkeys, and even ducks are eating soy, corn, and other assorted items when they should be eating grass, earthworms, and bugs.

Because of how we feed these animals, the typical chicken breast today has only 63 percent as much protein but 223 percent more fat than the chicken breasts I ate as a child forty years ago. And because of their diet, these chickens' fat is mostly the pro-inflammatory omega-6 type. This is the number one source of omega-6 fatty acids in people's diets today. In fact, 10 percent of the omega-6 we get from our diet is from chicken.

Fish

I am not sure if you have ever been to a fish farm, but they may be the worst of the lot of commercially raised animals. The last time I visited a fish farm, not only did the conditions smell horrible, but the fish didn't even look healthy. In fact, when you peeked into the tanks, the fish barely moved. I thought they were dead at first until one turned onto its side—when do fish lie on their sides? The water was brown and putrid looking with detritus along the surface. It cannot possibly be healthy to be consuming fish swimming in its own excrement. Even fish are what they eat.

You should be eating only wild, line-caught fish. Now, the debate about which type of fish can rage on. I'm not going to weigh in on that choice since by the time this book is published, the endangered list will have changed. My recommendation would be to check which fish aren't being overfished and then choose the wild varieties of that fish. You may want to check out this website from the folks at the Monterrey Bay Aquarium to see which fish are okay to eat this week: seafoodwatch.org.

Here's a quick guide for buying fish:

1. Buy it whole. Check to make sure the eyes are clear and not cloudy and the gills are bright red and not brown. This ensures that you've found a fish caught recently and stored properly.

2. When buying fillets, they should be firm to the touch and have an iridescent sheen, not dull. Oh, and ask to smell them—they should smell clean, not fishy.

3. Shellfish should be alive. Oysters should be closed, and clams and mussels closed or partly opened. (I remember driving home from the Hamptons as a small boy and stopping at the side of the road to buy these by the bushel, and my mother examining each one.) When the shell is partly opened, it should close if you tap it. Also, if you're buying shellfish in bags, which is much more common these days, there should be a date of harvest stamped on it—it's required by law.

IS MEAT CARCINOGENIC?

It all depends on who you ask! But any higher-protein diet book needs to reassure you that not only will you lose weight, you will be doing it in a healthy fashion. The World Health Organization (WHO) thinks meat will kill you. The reason they think this is because they put together a team of scientists to do a literature review of more than eight hundred studies that looked at the association between red meat and cancer.

They concluded that eating 50 grams of processed red meat a day—roughly one hot dog or six slices of bacon—raises your chances of getting colorectal cancer by 18 percent. They also concluded that beef, lamb, or pork is just as dangerous, although harder to quantify. So the WHO added processed meat to its Group 1 list of known carcinogens along with the likes of plutonium, cigarettes, radon, and sunshine, to name a few. Red meat was added to their Group 2A list of probable carcinogens. That list includes DDT (yeah, that doesn't cause cancer), lead, chemotherapy agents, and mustard gas.

Now that we can acknowledge that the WHO may be a little overzealous, let's look at the numbers a little more closely. Currently, five out of every one hundred of us will get colon cancer no matter what we eat. If everyone ate processed meat every day, that would increase the risk by 18 percent, to six in every hundred people. That's a very small increase and clearly doesn't warrant placing processed meat on the list of carcinogens. Living should be on that list at this rate. This isn't to say you may feel free to eat all the processed meat you want. A rare dalliance in processed organic meats is likely not that bad. Otherwise, steer clear.

Further, this list doesn't take into account the actual chances of getting cancer. The risk from eating meat is infinitesimal compared to, say, plutonium, where if you inhale the stuff you're pretty much guaranteed to get cancer and die. Yet they're on the same list.

These surveys also don't take into account those who ate healthfully and those who didn't. If you are the type of person who is overweight, smokes, and is sedentary, your unhealthy lifestyle is likely to cause cancer whether you eat meat or not—and chances are you eat processed meats and other foods.

Let's face another fact: Millions of years of evolution primed our muscles to thrive on animal protein, which means there is nothing inherently carcinogenic about meat consumed in modest amounts. If there were, our species would have died out long ago.

In 2012, the *American Journal of Clinical Nutrition* published an article called "Is Everything We Eat Associated with Cancer?" Of the fifty ingredients that the authors looked at, forty of them had been linked to cancer in one study or another.

My advice is to go ahead and enjoy red meat in moderation. The A-List Diet takes all of this into account when I prepared the menu plans, but if you want to make your own (and I thoroughly encourage you to do so), here are some things to keep in mind about meat:

1. Cook meat below temperatures of 500°F—anything above this temperature causes the formation of carcinogenic

compounds known as heterocyclic amines (HCAs) and polycyclic aromatic hydrocarbons (PAHs).

2. Consume all meat at medium-rare (well-done quadruples the amount of HCAs and PAHs).
3. Cut off the blackened bits of the meat—those are the HCAs and PAHs.

There are also seasonings and side dishes that can help lower your risk for getting cancer. Just as HCAs and PAHs can cause genetic mutations (epigenetics) in your body, there are also substances that can inhibit mutations:

1. Marinate meat in dark beer (can reduce PAHs by half).
2. Use beef rubs that contain turmeric, garlic, onion, or rosemary (can reduce HCAs by 94 percent).
3. Eat cruciferous vegetables such as broccoli, Brussels sprouts, bok choy, and cabbage as side dishes along with meat. They contain compounds that have been shown in research to have significant cancer-fighting benefits.

SUGAR

If it were up to me, this would surely be on the carcinogenic list rather than red meat. It is just a plain and simple fact that sugar kills. It has been linked to six of the top ten leading causes of death in the United States, and no one attacks this substance with the same voracity that they do meat. I have written a great deal about the dangers of sugar, so I will try to summarize how I feel about this evil as concisely as I can. If you want, you can always read more about the dangers of sugar in my Reality Health Check e-newsletter or Logical Health Alternatives monthly newsletter (you can sign up for both at DrPescatore.com).

In a recent review published in the journal *Mayo Clinic Proceedings,* researchers point to added sugar—and high-fructose corn syrup in particular—as the number one driving force behind the massive pre-diabetes and diabetes epidemic sweeping through the United States. Perhaps even more disturbing, another study (funded by the National Institutes of Health, no less) found that high-fructose corn syrup nearly doubled the death rate.

Yet in the most recent dietary guidelines, set out by the U.S. Department of Agriculture, there was no mention of reducing high-fructose corn syrup in your diet. I will grant you that the powers that be are finally seeing sugar as an issue, especially in terms of added sugar in beverages (they are still afraid to tackle that age-old myth that fruit is healthy for us). The latest guidelines did say you should limit your "added" sugars, but it certainly didn't make front-page headlines like the "red meat kills" foolishness.

Food manufacturers have picked up on the fact that consumers are looking for less sugar, so they've simply gotten savvy about how they add it to their products. Often, they add several different kinds so that they appear lower on the ingredient list, giving consumers the illusion that there really isn't that much sugar in any one product.

Other Added Sugars

Sucrose and high-fructose corn syrup are the most common added sugars in most processed foods. But here are some others to look out for—and steer clear of:

brown sugar	honey	raw sugar
corn sweetener	invert sugar	sweeteners ending in "-ose" (dextrose, fructose, glucose, lactose, maltose, sucrose
corn syrup	malt sugar	sweeteners ending in "-ol" (maltitol, erythritol, etc.)
rice syrup	molasses	syrup
fruit juice concentrates		

One sweetener in particular that people have been tricked into believing is healthy is agave. Agave is marketed as a safe, natural sugar substitute, but don't buy it! (Literally.) The fact is, agave has even more fructose than the evil that is high-fructose corn syrup. Agave contains anywhere from 70 to 95 percent fructose. High-fructose corn syrup contains about 55 percent. You do the math.

SugarGate

Many news outlets have recently blown the lid off the illicit relationship between the sugar industry and the supposedly "unbiased" scientific community.

A researcher from the University of California, San Francisco (UCSF) recently discovered actual documents detailing bribes paid to scientists by the sugar industry, in an effort to coerce them to underplay sugar's association to heart disease and to point the finger at saturated fat instead. And these weren't recent dealings, either. These bribes go as far back as the late 1960s.

It's proof that for the last fifty years, dietary recommendations for heart disease prevention have been based on fraudulent research and that the sugar industry itself had a hand in shaping the useless guidelines mainstream physicians still cling to today.

It seems that back in 1967 the Sugar Association gave three Harvard scientists what would amount to $50,000 today in return for publishing a review on the associations between sugar, fat, and heart disease.

Just last year, it came out that one beverage corporation was dumping millions of industry dollars right into the pockets of any researchers that would assist them in discrediting the very real link between soda drinking and obesity. Not to mention reports that junk food manufacturers are bankrolling studies that conclude that kids who eat candy actually weigh less.

It's also worth noting that while the Harvard scientists named in this latest exposé are no longer living, one of them, Dr. Frederick J. Stare, became chairman of the nutrition department at Harvard University. Another, D. Mark Hegsted, eventually became the USDA's head of nutrition—where he actually assisted in drafting an early version of the U.S. dietary guidelines.

Warnings about the dangers of saturated fat continue to plague our government's dietary guidelines. And it's only been in recent years that influential groups like the American Heart Association and the World Health Organization have conceded that added sugar might play any role at all in raising heart disease risk.

Sugar Kills

How did the story about drinking one soda per day upping heart disease risk by a whopping 30 percent pass by unnoticed, whereas the one about processed meat increasing your risk for colon cancer by 18 percent made front-page headlines?

Why is it taking so long for Americans to wake up and realize the "food" they're eating is killing them? And, most importantly, when are people going to realize that unless we loosen ourselves from the stranglehold of Big Agribusiness and Big Pharma, we are *never* going to be healthy as a nation? To paraphrase one of my patients, the pharmaceutical companies have propaganda departments that specialize in misinformation.

Roughly 15 percent of the daily calorie intake of the average American adult comes from sugar added to processed food. A whopping 37 percent of it comes from sugar added to sweetened beverages like soda.

Now, let me throw in my newest "fun fact" about sugar: In 1822, the average American took five days to consume the amount of sugar a modern American consumes in just one twelve-ounce soda.

Even more shocking? On average, Americans now consume that much sugar every seven hours. And it's literally killing us.

So to all those "experts" who think "everything is okay in moderation": *No, it's not.* Heroin's not okay in moderation. And neither is sugar. And let's be honest, there's nothing moderate about sugar consumption in this country. There is widely ranging debate about how much sugar is acceptable in a healthy diet.

The Institute of Medicine thinks it's acceptable to get 25 percent of your total calories from added sugar. The WHO is sticking with 10 percent. And the American Heart Association has recently dropped their recommendations to 5 percent and 7.5 percent for women and men, respectively.

But I've got news for them: They're all wrong. Because the only safe amount of added sugar in your diet is *none*. Which makes me wonder . . . am I the only doctor in this country that routinely counsels their patients on the harmful effects of sugar? Not a visit goes by where I don't ask each and every one of my patients about how their relationship with sugar has been since our last visit.

As I sat down to write this, a new study came out stating that the average child consumes their weight in sugar each year. That shocking statistic was all over the news and television when I happened to be passing through London, and I was so excited about it that I couldn't wait to get home and see what the American press was saying about it. Of course, by the time I landed a mere seven hours later, there wasn't so much as a mention in anything I was watching, reading, or listening to. You can read about the full details of that study in my Reality Health Check article "The UK Is Getting Serious about Restricting Sugar—Why Isn't the US?" at DrPescatore.com.

The Effects of Sugar on Your Body

1. **Waistline:** Since this is primarily a diet book, I thought I would start here. Any sugar, but particularly fructose, leads to a drop in energy at the cellular level, which leads to a slower metabolism, which leads to increased fat storage. Animals that hibernate tend to consume large amounts of fruit prior to hibernation to ensure they get enough fat to survive the winter. Sugar causes fat storage, not fat. If animals know this, and since we are supposedly the smartest animal on the planet, then why don't we? If we looked at nature more closely instead of ignoring it, we would probably be healthier for it.

2. **Heart:** People who get 25 percent or more of their calories from added sugar have a 275 percent higher chance of death from heart disease than those who get less than 10 percent.

3. **Pancreas:** According to research from around the world, all that sugar you consume increases your risk of developing diabetes by 26 percent.

4. **Brain:** When you eat sugar, your body turns off the production of orexin, which is a neurotransmitter that triggers wakefulness. This causes that brain fogginess and afternoon slump after eating lunch.

5. **Skin:** When your body digests sugar and processed foods, it bonds to collagen and elastin and results in glycation, forming harmful advanced glycation end products (AGEs). These are the worst kind of free radicals that wreak havoc throughout your body. High-fructose corn syrup causes ten times more glycation than ordinary glucose. Interestingly enough, rebuilding collagen requires amino acids— particularly, lysine—which you will get plenty of on the A-list program.

6. **Mood:** California State University did a study that showed that those who ate 24 grams of sugar in one sitting, which is the amount in a candy bar or a power bar (same thing, different packaging), had a quick energy spurt but an hour later reported less energy and a more stressful mood than beforehand. I know that many of you "stress eat," but do you really feel better after the initial high? No—simply switch to avocado or nuts for that quick energy relief. Trust me, it works, and you won't get the downside, nor will you feel guilty.

Sugar Addiction

Sugar has been shown to be every bit as addictive as cocaine or morphine, and the reward center of our brain is in constant overdrive because of the amounts we eat of refined and processed foods that contain high amounts of sugar. One in five Americans are believed to be sugar addicts.

Of the 40,000 items in the average American grocery store, 77 percent contain added sugars. We can control this, but we don't. We can legislate and force food manufacturers to change, but we don't. We try and are thwarted at every turn. Creating an addict is a perfect business model for businesses that sell food, but *we* end up paying the consequences.

The biggest problem facing the government, food manufacturers, and you, the dieter, is that reducing sugar and processed foods isn't enough, because moderation doesn't work with addiction. You would never allow a smoker to have just one cigarette or an alcoholic to have just one drink, yet you would encourage your friend or family member to have just one bite of your dessert. "One bite won't kill you," as they say. Well, perhaps it will.

I used to "blame" people for being overweight because they couldn't control what they ate. I now know I was wrong. Public policies were formed from bad science during the dark ages of "low fat." The public was told to not eat fat and to fear it. When fat is removed from a food, you need sugar to take its place or it isn't going to taste right. This led food manufacturers to add sugar to thousands of products and created a nation of addicts. We now know that this serious blunder led to the soaring rates of obesity, heart disease, diabetes, and cancer. Which is the perfect segue into discussing fats.

FATS

Let me start this section by revealing a truth that may shock you:

Fat has never been our enemy. Fat doesn't make you fat and sick. That honor has *always* gone to sugar.

Fat is important for our health and for the A-List Diet to work so efficiently. We need fat to make brain cells, keep our joints cushioned, synthesize vitamins, and keep us satiated so we don't overeat. I learned this critical lesson from the best of the best—Dr. Robert Atkins. And ever since then, I've been a "fat pioneer," extolling the virtues of fat and exposing sugar as the real culprit behind today's healthcare crisis.

Of course, not all fats are created equal. Some of them have extraordinary potential for not just promoting health but actually fighting disease. But others do the exact opposite. This is where mainstream "fat-phobic" advice has fallen short for years—they don't differentiate. But the research isn't letting us bury our heads in the low-fat sand any longer.

Healthy fats couldn't be more important to our health. Incorporating healthy fat with the right combination of amino acids will improve your feeling of fullness and satisfaction, provide fuel, and promote optimal cellular repair. You can't make cells without fat. Fats are the precursors of cell messengers that mediate inflammation—a key component in the A-List Diet. Fat is critical for hormone production and for heart, brain, and nervous system function.

The Eight Classes of Fats

Some will kill you and some will keep you incredibly healthy—and probably save your life.

1.   **Monounsaturated fatty acids (MUFAs)** are the healthiest kind of fat you can eat, according to research. Not only are they anti-inflammatory, but they also keep your blood lipids (cholesterol, triglycerides) healthy, help balance your blood sugar, and even help cut visceral fat by up to 20 percent. MUFAs are found in olives and olive oil, nuts and nut oils, and avocados. My favorite source is macadamia nut oil, which contains a greater percentage of MUFAs than the highest-quality olive oil.

2.   **Omega-3 fatty acids** are anti-inflammatory polyunsaturated fatty acids (PUFAs, see #4 below) and are found in fish oil, cold-water fish, walnuts, flaxseed, and chia seeds. They aid in controlling hunger, turning off your fat

genes, controlling blood sugar, and upping your metabolism.
They have also been shown to aid in reducing cholesterol
and preventing arthritis, asthma, ADHD, dementia, and
even depression.

3. **Medium-chain triglycerides** are an important fat-burning
tool and can help speed up your metabolism. These are
found in butter and coconut oil.

4. **Polyunsaturated fatty acids (PUFAs)** are a group of about
eighteen different kinds of fatty acids. Some are healthy
(like the omega-3s mentioned above) and some aren't (like
canola oil; see #6 below). The good ones can provide the
energy-producing mitochondria of your cells with fatty
acids that support metabolic efficiency.

5. **Trans-fatty acids** are the worst fats the world has ever seen,
and they have been in our food supply for decades—even
after science discovered they are deadly. They are manmade,
and our intestinal bacteria can't digest these foods, so they
end up lining our livers and arterial cell walls, causing death
and disease. These are also known as partially hydrogenated
vegetable oils, and are found in margarine and other butter
substitutes.

6. **Omega-6 fatty acids** are pro-inflammatory and are
abundant in processed foods, most cooking oils (including
canola), and pretty much every food you eat unless it is
organic. These are also PUFAs, but the bad ones. Up to 90
percent of the omega-6 in our diet comes from linoleic acid,
which promotes inflammation and fat storage. I'm sure
you are very familiar with some of these foods: grain-based
desserts, salad dressings, potato chips, corn chips, pizza,
pasta, and popcorn to name a few.

7. **Omega-9 fatty acids** are the neutral oils that do not lead
to inflammation and are healthy to consume. The biggest

food sources of these are: olives, macadamia nuts, avocados, almonds, pecans, and cashews.

8. **Saturated fats**—more on these later.

A Quick Word on Vegetable Oils

In a study conducted at the University of California, Riverside, mice were fed a series of four diets that contained about 40 percent fat—similar to the diet of most Americans. Of the four diets, one used coconut oil (pure saturated fat) and another used half coconut oil and half soybean oil (a vegetable oil). Mice on the half soybean oil diet showed weight gain, larger fat deposits, liver damage, diabetes, and insulin resistance. What are most Americans suffering from? Those same things. Those mice also gained 25 percent more weight than those on the coconut oil diet and 9 percent more than those on a sugar-enhanced diet. I guess one can say that soybean oil is 2.5 times more fattening than sugar.

Most of the vegetable oil used in processed foods and in restaurants is soybean oil. Soybean oil, like most vegetable oils, is almost all linoleic acid. Linoleic acid is an endocrine disruptor and wreaks havoc on our hunger hormones. Consuming vegetable oils in excess produces too much of the type of endocannabinoids, which tell the brain we are hungry. The THC in marijuana operates in much the same way to make you hungry.

According to a study in the *American Journal of Clinical Nutrition,* our per-capita consumption of soybean oil increased by more than 1,000 percent between 1909 and 1999. Today it is the fourth-largest contributor to our caloric intake. Corn and safflower oil are also hazardous to our health, but what makes soy so insidious is that it contains chemicals like genistein and daidzein that are estrogenic and disrupt hormones. I don't want to go too deeply into the dangers of soy—just suffice it to say that soy is the most damaged crop in this country, and you should avoid it like the plague.

Saturated Fats

Saturated fats get more of a bum rap than they deserve. This type of fat is found primarily in animal products—butter, cheese, and meat. And plenty of research has emerged in just the last couple of years proving that saturated fat isn't the problem the mainstream "experts" have made it out to be.

The only time saturated fat becomes really dangerous is when it's combined with sugar and refined flour to produce all those packaged, processed foods you find in the supermarket snack aisle and in fast food restaurants.

As long as you're getting your saturated fat from organic, grass-fed, grass-finished, minimally processed sources, it's perfectly okay to eat in moderation. In fact, I would go so far as to say it is a health food. Most of your fat intake should come from the protein and amino acids you eat. The rest will come from nuts, avocado, fish, and oils. If you get the majority of your protein from wild, hormone- and antibiotic-free animal foods such as eggs, salmon, chicken, grass-finished beef, and pasture-raised butter, you will get the essential monounsaturated and saturated fats you need in the right ratios.

And let's not forget that beef is not just one big saturated fat. About 50 percent of the fat in beef is unsaturated—the kind that we are being told to eat (but not from cows). Maybe not from commercially raised cows, but from happy, well-fed cows.

DAIRY

Dairy is also a saturated fat and has suffered from the ravages of the war against fat. The same rules of thumb apply to dairy as well as any protein drinks you may use: The source must be cows, sheep, goats, or even yaks that were fed and raised how they were supposed to be raised—that is, without antibiotics and growth hormones. I want to be clear here—when I mention dairy, I am talking about cheese or butter. I don't recommend yogurt (even the unsweetened ones) or milk.

In a very important study for the A-list crowd—and I mean all of you—when soy was compared to dairy, full-fat dairy won hands down. It resulted in a more sustained branched-chain amino acid (BCAA) concentration. That means the amino acids—the building blocks for protein—stayed in the body longer and the body was able to utilize them more. In other words, dairy did a better job at preserving and building muscle mass, which helps keep you stronger longer. Dairy is a natural source of these all-important BCAAs that you find in your protein boost shots and protein booster shakes.

And in another great study, cheese has been linked to a faster metabolism, reduced obesity, and—thanks to that—potentially a longer life. The lead researcher, a food scientist in Denmark, analyzed urine and fecal samples from fifteen men whose diets either contained cheese and milk or contained butter with no other dairy products. The findings: Those in the cheese group had higher levels of butyric acid, a gut microbe and short chain fatty acid that has been linked to lower obesity and faster metabolism.

In a fitting way to sum it all up, a University of Cambridge study raised some very important questions about the link between saturated fats and heart disease. In this meta-analysis of seventy-two different studies, researchers found that total saturated fat consumption was not linked to coronary heart disease. What will the powers that be do with that information?

CARBOHYDRATES

Although most people lump these all into one big group, all carbs are not created equal. My preferred carbohydrate sources for those on the A-list program are the carbohydrates that come in the form of vegetables. I can't tell you how many people forget that vegetables are carbohydrates. They are. Therefore, the A-List Diet is not a restricted-carbohydrate program; it is a program that limits you to healthy carbohydrates, such as vegetables, nuts, seeds, and some fruits.

VEGETABLES

A whopping 90 percent of adults in the United States fail to eat the daily recommended amount of vegetables. I have found that the trouble with getting Americans to eat enough vegetables is that we don't know how to cook them. And that's not to rehash the debate over stir-frying versus roasting versus steaming. The point is we have such a limited repertoire when it comes to vegetables, and that is what we have to change. There are so many vegetables that you probably aren't familiar with, but the A-List Diet is going to change that for you. Let's face it—who ever thought kale would become trendy?

There are plenty of vegetables in the A-list program, some specifically for the weight loss part of the program and then others for the weight maintenance portion. So, why do I prefer this source of carbohydrate? If you believe the American Diabetes Association, all carbohydrates are considered the same, but if you have been paying attention, you know that the type of carbohydrate (or the type of any food) you put into your body matters. So of course the same is true for vegetables.

Plants produce an arsenal of compounds to protect themselves from their natural enemies, and these compounds just happen to be good for us. Take broccoli and other cruciferous veggies, for example. These plants are packed with disease-fighting antioxidants. They also contain phytochemicals like sulforaphane and diindolylmethane (DIM), which help balance estrogen in the body and kill cancer cells. As you learned from the discussion of the different dieting types, any time you can keep your hormones balanced and in check, you will be able to lose weight more easily.

One recent three-year study showed that women who ate the most cruciferous veggies enjoyed a 35 percent lower risk of breast cancer recurrence. Even more impressively, they benefited from a 62 percent lower risk of dying from breast cancer—or dying from any cause at all, for that matter. Prospective studies performed with tens of thousands of participants have linked the consumption of cruciferous vegetables to reductions of approximately 50 percent in both bladder and prostate cancer and to a 30 percent drop in lung cancer.

Some studies suggest that as little as ½ cup of kale, broccoli, Brussels sprouts, or cauliflower a day could have a significant impact on your cancer risk. Chopping cruciferous vegetables and allowing them to sit for a few minutes before preparation is also important. This allows cancer-fighting phytochemicals to convert to more potent and bioavailable active forms, which means you'll be gobbling up more cancer protection with every bite.

Leafy greens are a big part of the A-list program—not because they fill you up with very little calories (remember, I don't care much for calorie counting) but because they, too, have health properties. Studies show that the consumption of leafy green vegetables—which contain generous amounts of dietary folate—can reduce the risk for pancreatic cancer by approximately 75 percent. You can get ample folate with a few hearty servings of spinach and avocado.

While we are on the subject of vegetables, I have to talk about America's favorite vegetables: French fries and ketchup. Data from the USDA shows that potatoes account for one-third of all vegetables Americans eat, and tomatoes are one-fifth. That means these two faux "vegetables" make up nearly *half* of the total vegetable intake for most people in this country. I say faux vegetables because potatoes are mostly starch and tomatoes are really a fruit.

According to the USDA, during the 2000s the "US per capita use of frozen potatoes averaged 55 pounds per year—42 pounds for fresh potatoes, 17 pounds for potato chips, and 14 pounds for dehydrated products." That's 128 pounds per person per year—of just potatoes!

And the impact ketchup has had is similarly frightening. In fact, ketchup accounts for roughly 15 percent of all tomatoes consumed in the United States. And the worst part is that ketchup is mostly sugar or high-fructose corn syrup. In fact, certain brands of ketchup contain much more sugar than ice cream.

GRAINS

Coming from an Italian family, I know that the next thing I am about to say borders on sacrilegious, but I don't think grains have a place in our diets. Simply stated, consuming grains of any kind can lead to health hazards, and this is especially true for those of us who have ever suffered from a weight problem.

I don't need to reinforce how you shouldn't be eating any white or refined grains—bread, pasta, cereals, cakes, cookies, and so on. I also don't think any grains with gluten have a place in our diet because of the high levels of inflammation they create. Many diet books have focused on this, and I am not going to dwell on it. However, we ought to take a look at whole grains, since many people still presume these to be a health food.

Whole Grains

Just because bread is brown doesn't make it a whole grain. Whole grains consist of the entire grain seed, usually referred to as the kernel. The kernel has three components: the bran, the germ, and the endosperm. Refined grains have neither the bran nor the germ, which means that most of the B vitamins and certain minerals and fiber have been stripped from the food product.

Food manufacturers don't make things any easier for us as they use terms in the packaging like multigrain, cracked wheat, seven-grain, 100 percent wheat, pumpernickel, and rye—and these are seldom whole grains at all. The fact is that food labels lie.

Some true whole grains include wheat berries, bulgur wheat, whole oats, whole rye, barley, buckwheat (kasha or buckwheat groats), whole corn, brown rice, and whole-grain wild rice. Other less-familiar whole grains are grano, farro, kamut, quinoa, amaranth, millet, sorghum, spelt, teff, freekeh, einkorn, red fife, and triticale.

Grains of any kind aren't that healthy and aren't really meant for human consumption, much less in the amount that most Americans eat them. Humans have been eating grains for some time, but it wasn't until the past hundred years that they became a larger staple of the American diet. We only started to really devour them in the 1950s, and by then they were overly processed and becoming farther and farther away from what our ancient ancestors first consumed, down to the actual grain itself being genetically engineered. Our bodies aren't evolutionarily prepared for eating the amount of grains that we eat, and we're certainly not ready to be eating these grains in their current genetically modified state. Let me remind you that wheat, corn, and soy are all mostly genetically modified. And we do not know the health implications that may have in the long run. If you really want to be healthy, stick to foods that don't require labeling in the first place.

If you think I'm crazy, I would like to draw your attention to a couple of particularly noteworthy characteristics of the modern wheat crop. Then you can decide for yourself whether this staple of the Standard American Diet is really something you should be eating.

Today's wheat has been hybridized (genetically modified) beyond all recognition, making it a far cry from the original heritage grains we consumed many years ago. They're shorter, higher-yield crops—which serves an obvious purpose. But they also contain more of a rapidly digested starch called amylopectin A. Higher amounts of amylopectin A mean that modern wheat—yes, even supposedly "healthy" whole wheat—hijacks your blood sugar more violently than heritage varieties from centuries ago. But that's only one part of the problem.

Wheat also contains gliadin, a component of gluten. If not properly digested, gliadin generates polypeptides that research suggests may induce a drug-like euphoria, acting as an opioid on the human brain. (Other noteworthy opioids include heroin, morphine, and oxycodone, just to name a few.)

In fact, studies as far back as the 1980s showed that treating subjects with naloxone reduced consumption of wheat at subsequent meals by as much as 28 percent. (Naloxone is a drug that reverses the effects of opiate drugs by binding with opioid receptors.) Is it any wonder we are obsessed with bread?

Grains Kill

So, before we leave the topic of grains, let's look at what the science tells us about eating these foods and the effects they have on our bodies.

One study looked at more than 1,200 normal, healthy adults between the ages of seventy and eighty-nine. According to the researchers, dementia risk was almost twice as high in participants who ate the most carbohydrates. It was similarly high in participants with the highest sugar intake. Yet the risk for mild cognitive impairment was 42 percent lower in people with the highest fat intake. And those who ate the most protein lowered their risk by 21 percent.

Simple carbohydrates have also been linked to prostate cancer in men. Swedish researchers specifically noted a correlation between elevated prostate cancer risk and higher consumption of refined carbohydrates or "white foods." Think low-fiber cereals, cakes, rice, and pasta. High intake of sugar-sweetened beverages—ahem, soda—was also associated with increased risk of prostate cancer, too.

LEGUMES

This is the group of foods that includes beans, lentils, peanuts, peas, and chickpeas, to name a few. Like all foods, legumes have a bright side and a dark side. And working them into your diet is largely a matter of balance.

First, the good news: Legumes are rich in fiber and protein. They're packed with nutrients like B vitamins, iron, potassium, and magnesium. They're low on the glycemic index scale. And they're also very cheap. The downside is that they all have relatively high carbohydrate counts. Luckily, legumes deliver complex carbohydrates, which means they take more time to digest, keep you full longer, and are easier on your blood sugar.

NUTS AND SEEDS

These are an unequivocal health food. Granted, they must be eaten in moderation, but there is no doubt that they are good for you and will play a very big role in the A-List Diet.

A new review published in the journal *PLOS ONE* found that a couple of handfuls of tree nuts a day may improve glycemic control in patients with type 2 diabetes. In addition, nuts can offer a variety of other health benefits, including improving blood glucose control, lowering harmful LDL ("bad") cholesterol and triglycerides, raising HDL ("good") cholesterol, and lowering blood pressure. Tree nuts include almonds, Brazil nuts, cashews, hazelnuts, macadamia nuts, pecans, pine nuts, pistachios, and walnuts.

When the researchers pooled all the data, they found that eating about ½ cup of tree nuts per day helped reduce both HgbA1c and fasting glucose levels over the course of around eight weeks.

It's also worth noting that some of the studies showing the most benefit investigated the effect of tree nuts as a dietary replacement for carbohydrates. Not only do tree nuts make a great, healthy replacement for carbs, they're also rich sources of magnesium and monounsaturated fat. And both of these nutrients have been linked to improved insulin sensitivity.

Researchers from the famous Nurses' Health Study (NHS) and NHS II, which followed over 137,000 women for roughly a decade, found that eating walnuts once a week was linked to a 13 percent lower risk of diabetes. And eating walnuts twice a week cut diabetes risk by 24 percent. Nuts have also been shown to slash cancer risk, and lower the risk of death—from *any* cause.

The bottom line: Nuts contain protein, fiber, minerals, vitamins, and antioxidants as well as good, healthy fats. And eating ½ cup each day will help keep your stomach full, your heart healthy, and your blood sugar balanced.

FRUITS

One of my long-time patients who always struggled with the rigors of dieting announced recently that she was finally going to stop eating bread and give up refined sugar for good. And I couldn't have been more pleased to hear it. But then she mentioned that in lieu of eating ice cream or cookies, she turned to dried fruit—like cranberries, pineapple, and figs—as "healthy" alternatives to sweets instead. Don't be fooled, the sugar content of dried fruit is staggering.

This person's concern was that limiting fruit would deprive her body of the glucose she needs to power her muscles and brain. That's a fair concern to have. But fruit isn't the only source of this critical fuel: Your body can break down any food you eat into glucose.

In fact, vegetables are actually a better source of glucose than fruit. Your body breaks down vegetables much more slowly than it breaks down fruit and other simple carbs. This means your brain and muscles get a steady supply of fuel, rather than the quick spike—and crash—that high-sugar foods (including fruits) provide.

It's the same principle behind avoiding fruit juice. Because when it comes down to it, there's a big difference between how your body processes a fresh apple and how it processes a glass of apple juice (which delivers the sugar content of multiple apples without any of the fiber or phytonutrients).

A team of Harvard researchers looked at data from three famous cohorts—the NHS, the NHS II, and the Health Professionals Follow-Up Study. The study, published in the *British Medical Journal,* showed that eating at least two servings of fruit every week lowered subjects' risk of developing diabetes by as much as 23 percent. On the other hand, those who drank one or more servings of fruit juice every day were as much as 21 percent more likely to wind up with diabetes. Think about that if you don't want to give up your glass of OJ in the mornings.

Fresh fruits play a role in a healthy diet because they are invaluable sources of antioxidants and phytochemicals that fight free radicals and help prevent chronic diseases. However, they are not as important as vegetables or as healthy since they contain a lot of sugar, which can counterbalance the important phytochemicals. For this reason, fruits are meant to be eaten in moderation as part of the A-list program.

One final tip: Fresh, in-season, locally grown fruits will always taste better than anything you can buy in the supermarket. So find the nearest produce stand or farmers' market and stock up!

THE SCIENCE SUPPORTING HIGHER-PROTEIN DIETS

Financed by the National Institutes of Health and published in the *Annals of Internal Medicine*, a new study included a racially diverse group of 150 men and women—a rarity in clinical nutrition studies. The participants were assigned to follow either a diet that limited carbs or a diet that limited fat for one year. Neither diet limited overall calories. Results showed that people who avoided carbohydrates and ate more fat—even saturated fat—lost more body fat and had fewer cardiovascular risks than people who followed the low-fat, carb-heavy diet that health authorities have blindly favored for decades.

By the end of the yearlong trial, people in the low-carb group had lost an average of eight pounds more than those in the low-fat group. They had significantly greater reductions in body fat than the low-fat group, and more improvements in lean muscle mass. And they enjoyed these benefits despite the fact that neither group changed their physical activity levels. And the low-fat group appeared to lose more muscle than fat. And that's what kills your metabolism.

It's also worth noting that the people in the low-carb group took in a little more than 13 percent of their daily calories from saturated fat, which is more than double the limit recommended by the American Heart Association. But the majority of their fat intake was unsaturated fats, like avocado and macadamia nut oil.

In the end, people in the low-carbohydrate group saw markers of inflammation and triglycerides plunge. Their HDL ("good") cholesterol rose more sharply than it did for people in the low-fat group. In fact, they ultimately did so well that they managed to lower their Framingham risk scores, which calculate the likelihood of a heart attack within the next ten years. Meanwhile, the low-fat group on average had no improvement in their scores.

These results make sense when you consider that eating refined carbohydrates tends to raise the overall number of LDL ("bad") cholesterol particles and shift them toward the small, dense variety, which contributes to atherosclerosis. In contrast, saturated fat tends to make LDL particles larger, more buoyant, and less likely to clog arteries—at least when carbohydrate intake remains low.

Hopefully, this study can put an end to the misinformation, once and for all, because it showed that low-carb diets don't contribute to endothelial dysfunction or vascular stiffness—two risk factors behind high blood pressure and plaque formation.

CHAPTER EIGHT

Fitness Prescription

There are many studies proving the weight-loss and health-enhancing benefits of exercise. You simply can't afford to miss out on all the amazing things that exercise can do for you. I know that it may be hard to change how you eat and start exercising all at the same time, but I am not asking for a lot of exercise. For instance, one study tells us that those who jog the least have more cardiovascular benefits than those who jog moderately or those who jog the most—who knew?! See how much fun exercise myth-busting facts can be? I hope this will encourage you to get off your seat.

Believe me, I have heard all the excuses. But I'll tell you what I tell my patients:

1. Start with something—I don't care which form of exercise you choose.
2. Carve out a time in your schedule to get it done. Even if that means getting up earlier than usual, using some of your lunch break, or doing it immediately after work.
3. Treat exercise the same way you would treat any professional obligation you have. Because it is every bit as important (if not a whole lot more).

I believe in exercise so much that I have incorporated a medical fitness facility right in my office, complete with a medical exercise specialist to make sure my patients are getting the exercise they need in a safe, well-monitored environment.

All my celebrity clients incorporate exercise into their A-List Diet regimen. You can't avoid this part. Exercise increases longevity and decreases your risk of heart disease, diabetes, strokes, cancer, bone loss—you name it. Just like good food, physical activity is a fundamental cornerstone of lasting health. Yet fewer than 5 percent of American adults get even thirty minutes of moderate-intensity exercise on a weekly basis.

SITTING DISEASE

This condition is very real. And it's deadly, too. If you're an older woman who sits for more than eleven hours every day—whether it's in front of the TV or behind a desk—you're 12 percent more likely to die early. You're also 21 percent more likely to die of cancer, and as much as 27 percent more likely to die of heart disease.

This unsettling discovery comes courtesy of a brand-new study of 93,000 postmenopausal American women. Not too long ago, researchers reviewed more than two hundred cancer studies from around the world. Sedentary lifestyle—or as I call it, sitting disease—was linked to nearly 49,000 cases of breast cancer and 43,000 cases of colon cancer.

It's also been shown that sitting for more than three hours per day can cut your lifespan by two years. And watching TV for more than two hours a day results in losing another year and a half. Exact numbers vary, but the general consensus is that more than three to six hours of sitting per day—regardless of your exercise routine—is the deadly tipping point.

Sit Less

If you want a longer and healthier life:

1. Simply get up out of your seat.
2. Take regular, short walks to break up your day.

3. Commute by walking or biking as often as you can.
4. Park farther away from your destination.
5. Get off the bus/subway one stop earlier and walk the rest of the way.
6. Work at your desk while standing up.

When you get home:

1. Don't set up camp on the couch.
2. Get in the kitchen and cook up a delicious meal.
3. Take a nice walk around the block after dinner.
4. Don't sit for more than a couple of hours at a time. If you have to, set a timer. When it beeps, get up and do something. Anything. Make it a habit and you'll add three years to your life.

Studies show that simply by walking to work, you can cut your risk of diabetes by 40 percent and your risk of high blood pressure by nearly 20 percent. Meanwhile, for every twenty-minute walk you squeeze into your day, you'll cut your risk of heart disease by 8 percent.

I give almost all my patients a prescription for exercise, just as I would for any other part of their treatment plan. However, I'm not naive to the fact that people hate to exercise. In fact, I'd be willing to bet most of my patients would say it's the hardest recommendation I give them.

I'm not going to lay out a full exercise plan here because it's important to work with a skilled professional who can help you tailor an exercise regimen for your particular needs. I understand my readers have different backgrounds in terms of age, level of activity, level of infirmity, and so on. The fact is there is no one-size-fits-all approach.

Don't forget—exercise doesn't always have to "feel" like exercise. Gardening, bowling, golfing, ballroom dancing . . . all these hobbies get you moving—without a gym membership. Whenever you can, add activity to your day. Wash the car, play hide-and-seek with your kids or grandchildren, get in a game of ping-pong, anything.

EXERCISE 101

A combination of aerobic and resistance training is pretty universally recommended these days, even by the troglodytes responsible for the federal government's health guidelines. Current US guidelines suggest 150 minutes of moderate physical activity per week.

This sounds like a lot. But for practical purposes, that's roughly twenty minutes a day. And a typical moderate-intensity exercise would be walking at a pace of about 3 miles per hour. If you've ever used a treadmill, you'd recognize that as pretty slow. It's a pace that would get you knocked down on a New York City sidewalk.

Aerobic activities include such things as running, using the elliptical machine, biking, playing tennis, rowing, stair climbing—basically any activity that raises your heart rate. To find your maximum heart rate, subtract your age from 220. The resulting number is the highest your heart rate should ever go in beats per minute. For example, if you're fifty years old, then the highest heart rate you should hit is 170 beats per minute. You generally want to keep your heart rate at 85 percent of your max. (In the above example, that would be 145 beats per minute.) This maximizes your body's oxygen consumption and lowers your heart rate when you're at rest and maximizes fat burning. I like to see my patients do at least fifteen minutes of aerobic activity each day.

Resistance training includes weight lifting, exercise bands, yoga, and Pilates. (Some may argue that yoga and Pilates are not true resistance activities, but they do increase muscle tone by using the weight of your body, so I include them in this category.) Resistance exercise boosts your strength and your muscle mass, while upping your metabolism and cutting down body fat.

I prefer strength training over other types of exercise because it offers the best of both worlds. You get your heart rate up while increasing muscle mass at the same time. A lot of women shy away from this type of exercise for fear of bulking up. But this is a myth. Women simply don't have the hormonal environment necessary to get really big without an extraordinary amount of work. Strength training, or a weight-resistance exercise program, helps build muscle mass, maintain bone mass, and improve metabolism. Aim for two or three times a week, about forty minutes each time.

Meanwhile, stretching exercises are necessary if you want to stay comfortable and mobile. These exercises maximize your range of motion. They also boost joint function, tendon flexibility, and muscle performance. That's why stretching is so effective when it comes to preventing and treating musculoskeletal injuries and for preventing falls. Basic stretching should be done daily. Simply do it while you're watching TV in the evenings!

Two recent studies published in the *Archives of Internal Medicine* found that aerobic and resistance training combined lowered diabetes risk by a whopping 59 percent. And here are some other statistics about moderate physical activity:

1. Reduced all-cause mortality by 38 percent
2. Reduced risk of heart disease death by 49 percent
3. Decreased basal insulin levels
4. Increased insulin sensitivity
5. Lowered HgbA1c levels, a measure of long-term blood-sugar control
6. Decreased diabetes risk by 34 percent

OTHER PROVEN HEALTH BENEFITS

I probably don't need to reiterate the fact that exercise affects your entire body, and I certainly won't bore you with the study details. Just know that I am not reporting on body-builder levels of exercise here—just moderate as described above. Here are some of the things that exercise has been proven to do:

1. Improve sexual functioning in men
2. Slow and even ward off cognitive decline and dementia
3. Increase the length of your telomeres
4. Decrease risk of stroke
5. Decrease risk of cancer
6. Decrease bone loss
7. Slow down the aging process
8. Decrease menopausal symptoms

From the results of all these studies, it certainly appears that exercise may be just the magic bullet you have been searching for.

OTHER EXERCISE TIPS TO HELP ENSURE SUCCESS

Before you begin exercising:

1. Talk to your doctor about any new exercise program.
2. Choose activities you enjoy so you'll stick with your workouts.
3. Find an exercise partner to help you stay motivated.
4. Buy supportive shoes—the right ones for your activity.
5. Pick a start date and start.
6. Be consistent.

After you begin exercising:

1. Allow at least ten minutes to warm up before starting to exercise rigorously. To do this, choose an activity that gently works major muscles.
2. Stretch the muscles that will absorb most of the shock of your exercise routine.
3. If you have any new pain while exercising, stop immediately—do not push through it—and let your doctor know.

4. Gradually boost the distance, length, or intensity of your workout.
5. Mix it up. Do different exercises to keep your mind from getting bored and to keep your body challenged.

DON'T EAT MORE

Unless you are a body builder or wish to increase muscle mass, most of us do not need to eat any more food when we exercise. Yes, it might make us hungrier, but you must not give in to the temptation or reward yourself for a job well done, because it takes a whole lot of running, walking, biking, or swimming to burn off that reward doughnut.

People tend to inflate the fat-burning power of their exercise regimen in a very real way. A quick run in the morning doesn't entitle you to a food reward—that's counterproductive to our goal here. Losing weight isn't always easy or comfortable. (And depending on your metabolism, neither is maintaining it.) I'm not trying to be a killjoy. That's just the way it is.

I'm not a gym rat by any stretch of the imagination. I was an overweight child and hated exercise with a passion. So I understand the intensity of the dislike. I still don't enjoy going, but I make regular exercise a core part of my life. Please join me. All it takes is practice and, most importantly, commitment.

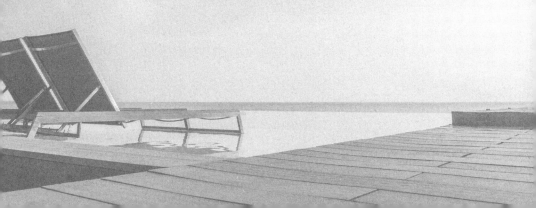

PHASE THREE

MAINTENANCE (FOR A LIFETIME)

CHAPTER NINE

More Food Recommendations

You've made it and you've reached your goal. Now what do you do? The biggest obstacle for any dieter is to figure out how to make dieting a way of life, not something you go on and go off. Diet must equal lifestyle. This chapter contains more lists and more details—the list of foods will grow, as will the complexity of your choices. Most dieters fail when they are given more choices, but with the A-List Diet, just stick to my guidelines and you'll succeed.

At this point in the program, the protein booster shakes and the protein boost shots have transformed your body into a lean, mean metabolic machine. By the end of the first thirty days, your level of inflammation will have been dramatically reduced. If you've reached your goal weight or are close to it, you are now primed for the reintroduction of a variety of foods. If you are not at your goal weight by thirty days, stick to phase two until you reach it.

PROTEINS

There are no new proteins to incorporate into your diet. Proteins are such a key component of the A-list program that you can eat all proteins right from the beginning of phase two, so just continue on your maintenance program eating about 1 gram of protein per pound of body weight each day. Keep in mind that you are now at a lower body weight, so adjust accordingly.

COMPLEX CARBOHYDRATES: VEGETABLES, LEGUMES, AND BEANS

beefsteak tomatoes	cherry tomatoes	grape tomatoes	green tomatoes
plum tomatoes	acorn squash	banana squash	buttercup squash
butternut squash	calabaza	delicata squash	golden nugget squash
hubbard squash	Japanese squash	pumpkin	sweet dumpling squash
turban squash	black-eyed peas	peas	scallop squash
chayote	black radishes	burdock root	black salsify
carrots	celery root	jicama	soy beans
daikon	horseradish root	lotus root	chickpeas
parsnip	rutabaga	salsify	turnip
sweet onion	wax gourd	sprouted beans	snow pea pods
snow peas	shelly beans	beer bean	edamame
cannellini beans	cranberry beans	fava beans	lima beans
mung beans	hyacinth beans	yellow beans	cow-eyed beans
chayote	chicory root	broad beans	water chestnut
beluga lentil	black chick pea	brown lentil	chana dal
chowli dal	French green lentil	horse gram lentil	masoor dal
moth sprouts	mung dal	toor dal	split black lentil
red lentil	black lentil	white lentil	split lablab beans
yellow lentil	sweet potato	yam	

You should slowly incorporate these foods back into your diet. I recommend ½ cup cooked twice per week for one month, then three times per week for the second month of maintenance; after that you must get a feel for how much you can eat. Each person is different, so there is no hard and fast rule. However, these foods will never be something that you can eat in unlimited quantities.

COMPLEX CARBOHYDRATES: LEGUMES AND TUBERS

arrowroot	cassava	Japanese artichoke	Jerusalem artichoke (sunchoke)
dasheen	malanga	white potatoes	new potatoes
red potatoes		taro	yucca
russet potato	fingerling potato	new potato	huckleberry potato
oca potato	purple potato	Idaho potato	yellow Finn potato
Yukon gold potato	boniato	tropical yam	Japanese yam
Okinawan purple potato	yamaimo	pigeon pea	yellow pea
garbanzo pea	green split pea	adzuki beans	anasazi beans
beets	black beans	breadfruit	corn
feijoa	great northern beans	red kidney beans	miso
moth bean	natty	navy beans	picante beans
pinto beans	pigeon beans	plantain	red beans
white beans			

This group of foods should be used sparingly and never while transitioning to the new A-list you. They should be consumed only once you have reached your goal weight and have stayed there for at least one month. Then you can eat these about twice per month, but again, please use your judgment; if you find yourself gaining weight, cut back; if maintaining, you are doing the right thing.

Beans and legumes should never be your primary source of protein and amino acids because they are simply incomplete. They are an inferior source of protein. Vegetarians of the world—good for you. I am not including a vegetarian program per se, but you can certainly choose from the foods that I have provided to ensure you get as much from the A-list program as you can. Please, if you insist on being a vegetarian, don't be a carbo-tarian, which is what most vegetarians in this country are. Eat vegetables, not breads and pasta.

GRAINS

This is actually not a recommended food category, because I don't think humans should be eating grains. However, if you insist on eating grains, here are the ones that I think are the healthiest:

1. **Freekeh** is an ancient Middle Eastern grain. It has a lower glycemic index than brown rice or quinoa and twice the fiber. It cooks the same way, and this green wheat is fire-roasted after harvesting to give it a slightly smoky taste. It is also higher in protein and amino acids.

2. **Ancient wheats** include such foods as einkorn, red fife, spelt, kamut, and farro. These haven't been genetically engineered and therefore are healthier.

3. **Amaranth** is high in protein, iron, and calcium.

4. **Quinoa** is packed with vitamins and minerals and is a complete protein as it contains all nine essential amino acids.

5. **Buckwheat** is a staple of the Japanese diet and is also known as soba. It is actually not a grain but a seed related to rhubarb. Most soba noodles sold in this country are mostly

wheat, so be sure to ask if you order soba out; and if you buy it to cook, please check the ingredients list.

6. **Barley** is high in vitamin B, selenium, and manganese.
7. **Millet** has high levels of iron, copper, manganese, phosphorous, and magnesium.
8. **Teff** is the world's smallest grain, so it's too hard to process all the goodness out of it. It is rich in protein and calcium, with a sweet, nutty flavor.

If you opt to include these, I would recommend in phase three only ½ to 1 cup cooked per week. If you are an active body builder, then you can increase that to every day that you work out. Be very careful with your grain amounts and you will be able to maintain the A-list gains that you've just made. Personally, I leave grains for special occasions.

DAIRY

plain unsweetened full-fat yogurt	kefir (unsweetened)	buttermilk	kumiss
jocoque	oat milk	fromage blanc	petit-suisse
quark	labneh		

These foods are sweeter than the other forms of dairy mentioned in phase two. Yogurt should be limited to once per week in the first month of phase three. Oat milk should be limited to 2 ounces each time you choose to drink it or use it for something. The cheeses should be limited to 1 ounce a couple of times per week while your body is adjusting to the new foods.

As with any food in phase three, the less you eat of these the easier it will be to maintain your weight. Remember that you have to be the judge of how much of these foods you can eat.

NUTS AND SEEDS

bread nut seeds	chestnuts	chufa	gingko nut
kluwak	kola nut	horned water chestnut	

During phase three, you can incorporate these food items up to 1 ounce per week if you desire.

FRUITS, PART I

½ apple	Asian pear	loquat	quince
Seckel pear	prickly pear	½ grapefruit	Meyer lemon
rangpur	tangelo	ugli fruit	kiwi
champagne grapes	aprium	tart cherries	donut peach
nectarine	peach	tangerine	green banana
pomegranate	green papaya	ackee	dragon fruit
kiwana	carissa	cashew apple	jujube
rambutan			

These fruits are still somewhat lower in sugar but not quite as low as the list in phase 2, so it's best to limit your intake to just a few times a week in phase three (and likely for the rest of your life).

FRUITS, PART II

cape gooseberries	baby kiwi	currants	figs
prunes	dried fruit of any kind	elderberries	jaboticaba
olallieberry	pear	bergamot orange	blood orange
Panama orange	pomelo	cedro	mandarin orange

apricot	sweet cherries	sour cherries	green almonds
red grape	green grape	banana - yellow	red banana
plantain	dates	figs	Kadota fig
mango	papaya	pineapple	atemoya
jackfruit	soursop	sapote	breadfruit
canistel	capulin cherry	toddy palm seeds	mangosteen
sapodilla	white sapote	mamey sapote	monstera
otaheite gooseberry	gooseberry	custard apple	durian

You may have something from this group of fruits a few times a month. These are some of the most common and popular fruits. Unfortunately, they also have the highest sugar contents. They should be reserved for occasional treats. This category may be eaten rarely or every once in a while but definitely not on a regular basis.

So, as you can see, you don't have to give up fruit. There are lots of options to choose from. They're nature's desserts, so go ahead—just opt for the healthier choices. But under no circumstances should you have fruit juice as the juice gives you all the sugar and none of the fiber and much less of the polyphenols.

CONDIMENTS

bean paste	black bean sauce	chili bean paste	dwenjang
hoisin sauce	hot bean paste	oyster sauce	red sweet bean paste
sweet bean paste	umeboshi puree	tomato paste	tomato sauce
Worcestershire sauce	chutney	mole	salsa
taco sauce	enchilada sauce	tamarind paste	

This group of condiments should be used sparingly since they contain sugar or are made from carbohydrates. A little of these go a long way.

MISCELLANEOUS AND ALCOHOL

fruit vinegars	sherry vinegar	verjus	dark rum
demerara rum	wine	beer	liqueurs
crème liqueurs	schnapps	champagne	brandy
apricot brandy	Armagnac	cachaça	cognac
framboise	fruit brandies	grappa	kirsch
Metaxa	pisco	plum brandy	sake

This category contains much larger amounts of sugar than those listed in phase two. I recommend caution when introducing these into your diet. Go slowly.

CHAPTER TEN

The A-List Guide to Conquering Food Addiction

I know no one likes to talk about this, but we can be just as addicted to food as we can be to any other "recognized" addictive substance like drugs, alcohol, and nicotine. It takes just three days to overcome your addiction to sugar and simple carbohydrates—hence the detox part of the A-List Diet.

Sadly, it is far easier to be unhealthy than to be healthy in this country, so I applaud you for the courage it has taken to even get to this point in the book. And just know that while the A-List Diet is going to work, it is going to work only if you work it, as they say. The A-List Diet will alleviate your physical cravings, break your food addictions, and help you control your addict-like behaviors.

But it won't completely eliminate that psychological "need" for the cookies, bread, and candy you once loved so much. The truth is, your brain may always want those foods. As I mentioned in chapter 1, to this day my favorite food is ice cream. And I will always look at the freezer section in grocery stores where the pints are kept to reassure myself that they haven't gone away and that my favorite flavors are still there. I just don't ever open the doors. I know that probably sounds bizarre. But right or wrong, we each have to find our own coping mechanisms. Whatever keeps you clean, so to speak.

Since many of us eat emotionally—that is, we eat with our minds and not our hunger mechanism—how do we push through this? Breaking this psychological cycle is every bit as important as breaking your physical dependence on certain types of food. But in this day and age, it is really difficult. I can look out the window of my office set nineteen floors above the streets of Manhattan and see twelve different places to buy lunch, and I wouldn't eat in any of them because not one of them serves anything that is even remotely healthy. So, what is it?

Is it our culture of gluttony at work? The limitless abundance of cheap, processed, nutrient-devoid junk food? Or maybe we simply have no self-control? I'm certainly not willing to take any of these factors off the table entirely. I think it's likely that they're all at play to some degree or another. That's why I'm skeptical of referring to obesity as a disease.

It's an understandable but problematic label, as far as I'm concerned. Not least of all because it has the potential to undermine the important role of personal accountability when it comes to maintaining a healthy weight.

I have the same reservations when it comes to the concept of food addiction. Find me a person who's addicted to broccoli, and I'll buy it wholesale. Until then, you have to admit that there's a whole lot of gray area here. That said, there's no denying the research. And quite a few studies have revealed that sugar lights up the same pleasure centers in your brain as cocaine and heroin.

A 2012 study on ice cream analyzed the effects of ice cream consumption on the brain—more specifically, the striatum, which is the brain's reward center. According to the researchers, milkshakes "robustly activated the striatal regions." (Translation: These subjects' reward centers lit up like it was the Fourth of July.)

But they also found that frequent ice cream consumption actually dulled this response. (Translation: You build a "tolerance" to it, requiring more and more to get the same satisfaction. Just as with drug addiction.)

But it's not just ice cream that causes problems. Recently, a team of scientists observed that Oreo cookies lit up even more neurons in rats' pleasure and reward centers than cocaine or morphine. (Believe it or not, the rats went straight for the cookie's middle, just like in the commercials.) All in all, the evidence is pretty damning for sugar.

So I don't think there can be much question that sugar is as alluring as hard drugs for a huge portion of the population. Factor in the natural mood swings that come with reactive hypoglycemia—better known as a "sugar crash"—and you've got a foolproof recipe for compulsive overeating.

At the end of the day, sugar is sugar is sugar. Too much of it is going to leave you fat, hungry, and hooked. So the next step should be clear: If you want to regain control over your weight, you have to kick your bad habits for good. It goes without saying that food addicts can't abstain from eating altogether, which is an argument I hear over and over again. But overcoming your addiction does require abstaining from certain "trigger foods." At all times.

Luckily, it takes only three days of being sugar-free to shake that insatiable hunger. Trust me: That urgent feeling of addiction goes away in just seventy-two hours. I've seen it happen with thousands of patients. The physiological craving breaks.

But that doesn't mean it will always be easy from then on out. It won't be, especially not in the beginning. Because then the psychological craving takes over and it becomes largely a mind-over-matter endeavor. And the first three days will be the hardest part of your journey, which is why I set up the detox part of the program. After that, I urge you to focus on the many foods you may eat instead.

There is a difference between craving and true hunger. And the farther you move away from your addiction to sugar and wheat, the clearer this distinction will be to you. Becoming an A-lister may be difficult at times. Our nation simply isn't set up to be healthy, so you will have extra work to do in order to overcome that. But it's not impossible. In fact, I've treated many patients who have successfully achieved those very goals of health and weight management.

We live in a time of abundance. We no longer eat out of necessity. We eat because we're angry, because we're sad, or just because the food's there. Our emotions almost always dictate how, what, and where we eat. And breaking this psychological dependence on food is every bit as important as any other part of a diet program.

THE LONG HAUL

Losing weight is the easiest part for most people and therefore I spend most of my time teaching people how to keep the weight off once they've lost it. It's not sexy and it's not the stuff people want to hear, but it is critical if you want to achieve your lifelong health and weight goals. Keeping weight off directly impacts just about every aspect of your health.

There are many reasons why you may be struggling with a weight issue. And the only way to truly take control of your weight is to look at all the reasons why it may be happening. That's why I included this chapter. You will be successful only if you are consistent and understand the potential pitfalls surrounding you.

What surprises my patients most about this phase of their journey to good health is that most of the "tips" are psychological in nature. The reason for this shift in focus is that by the time you've lost a significant amount of weight, you've already committed to eating a healthy diet and getting some exercise, so you don't need specific advice on what to eat or how to get moving.

But often people haven't necessarily addressed their underlying relationship with food, even if they've managed to shed twenty, thirty, forty pounds or more over and over again.

And that's one of the biggest mistakes you can make—excluding the mind from any weight loss plan will invariably lead to failure. In fact, a recent study published in the *Journal of the American Academy of Nurse Practitioners* pointed out various behavioral and emotional factors that lead to regaining weight. Here are some of the most important:

1. **Unrealistic expectations:** This is why I never set a specific weight loss goal with my patients. All weight loss is good—it doesn't matter how much or how long it takes, as long as the trend is down.

2. **Failure to achieve weight loss goals:** If you're frustrated and disappointed that you haven't reached some arbitrary number you had in your mind, you're much more likely to throw in the towel.

3. **Dichotomous (or "black and white") thinking:** People who think this way tend to have a hard time accepting anything less than their original goal. And when they can't reach it, they give up.

4. **Eating to regulate mood:** This is the biggest enemy of weight management. Find other ways to manage your emotions.

5. **Body image**: Individuals who were more satisfied with their appearance, and whose body image steadily improved throughout the time period studied, were more likely to maintain their weight loss. Be proud, and not afraid, of your new body.

As a recovering obese person, I have always been fascinated by the psychological components of eating. I firmly believe that unless you conquer your mind, you will never conquer your weight or health issues. It's just not going to happen. That's why my second book, *Thin for Good*, highlighted what I called the "eleven emotional levels of eating." I would bet that if you really thought about it, you've gone through each and every one of these emotions at some point:

1. Anger with the way you look and feel
2. Frustration at not being able to lose the weight fast enough—or at all

3. Sadness over losing your old way of life
4. Fear of the unknown and your changing body—of being thin or becoming fat again
5. Acceptance of the real reasons you are overweight or unhealthy
6. Trepidation about your new life as a thinner, healthier person
7. Envy toward people who have not struggled with their weight like you
8. Boredom with your new healthy eating habits
9. Relief over knowing that you have finally succeeded in meeting your weight loss goals
10. Joy from your sense of accomplishment and how good you look and feel
11. Contentment with your new body and lifestyle

Number 11 is the level of true self-acceptance and it's the scariest emotional level, by far. Recognizing this emotional journey will be one of the most important things you do in your quest to get healthy. Just remember that it's not something you need to do alone. In fact, I find that my patients with a strong support system in place achieve the greatest success.

So don't hesitate to seek out an experienced counselor or even a local support group. Overeaters Anonymous is a fantastic resource that can help connect you with other people who are also working to overcome addictive eating behaviors (visit OA.org to find a meeting near you). Recovery, in this case as with all others, truly is one day at a time.

CHAPTER ELEVEN

A-List Recipes

I sure hope everyone likes to cook as much as I do, because these recipes I've created for my A-listers are delicious. Sadly, cooking is becoming a lost art in this country as many of us look for quick and easy options. "Fast" food is always on our minds, yet spending thirty minutes preparing a healthy and nutritious meal is time well spent. Cooking is just another new habit to break in.

These recipes will bring you to the top of your A-list game, so I encourage you to be inventive: Swap out the proteins and the vegetables for something that you like better, that is more affordable to you, or that is more in line with your amino acid profile and your dieting type. Try something more alkaline that you like better.

A lot of these recipes can be made in one pot, though I threw in a few more complicated dishes for those of us who do like to cook. Many of the dishes I am recommending are made for at least four people. If you're only cooking for yourself, you can make one dish and have it last for several meals. But do try to make something different at least four days per week so you are rotating the all-important amino acids. Many of my patients will take a Saturday or a Sunday to cook so they have food ready for the week. You don't have to cook every day if you do this simple task on a weekend or whenever you may have some time. Plus, it's super fun to involve the entire family.

On to the recipes. Please enjoy!

Breakfast

Fried Egg and Bacon with Watercress

Serves 2

1 teaspoon macadamia nut oil, or more if needed
4 Canadian bacon slices
2 jumbo eggs
coarse salt and freshly ground black pepper
2 thin red onion slices
mayonnaise, to taste
1 cup watercress sprigs, tough stems removed

1. Heat the oil in a large cast-iron or nonstick skillet over medium-high heat. Add the bacon in a single layer and cook, flipping once, until warmed through, 2 to 3 minutes. Transfer to a plate and cover to keep warm.
2. Add more oil to the skillet if necessary and crack the eggs into the skillet. Season with salt and pepper and fry until the whites are set but the yolks are still runny, about 3 minutes.
3. To assemble, place an onion slice on each plate. Spread a little mayonnaise on the onion slices, then lay two bacon slices on top of each onion. Season with salt and pepper. Top each with some watercress and an egg and serve.

Fried Egg and Gruyère on a Bed of Avocado

Serves 2

1 avocado
1 tablespoon macadamia nut oil
½ teaspoon kosher salt
1½ teaspoons freshly squeezed lemon juice
2 eggs
coarse sea salt and freshly ground black pepper
Gruyère cheese
½ cup broccoli sprouts

1. In a medium bowl, mash together the avocado, oil, kosher salt, and lemon juice with a fork until it's chunky. Divide evenly between two plates.
2. Heat a nonstick sauté pan over medium-high heat. Crack the eggs into the skillet. Season with sea salt and pepper and fry until the whites are set but the yolks are still runny, about 3 minutes.
3. Just before the eggs are finished cooking, use a vegetable peeler to shave eight thin slices of Gruyère cheese onto the eggs, allowing some of the cheese to melt onto the pan and crisp up.
4. When the eggs are cooked and the cheese melted, carefully transfer one egg onto each bed of avocado. Top each with some broccoli sprouts and serve.

Mexican Fried Eggs

Serves 2

½ cup Mexican crema
1 tablespoon minced chipotles in adobo
3 teaspoons macadamia nut oil, or more if needed, divided
4 ounces fresh chorizo, removed from its casing
1 poblano chile, seeded and cut into ¼-inch-thick rounds (about 1 cup)
½ white onion, cut into ¼-inch-thick rounds (about 1 cup)
2 (½-inch-thick) eggplant slices
coarse sea salt and freshly ground black pepper
2 jumbo eggs
½ avocado, thinly sliced
chopped fresh purslane, for garnish

1. Stir together the crema and chipotle and set aside.
2. Heat 1 teaspoon of the oil in a cast-iron or nonstick skillet over medium heat. Add the chorizo and cook, stirring occasionally and breaking it up into bite-size pieces, until just cooked through and browned in places, 4 to 5 minutes. Using a slotted spoon, transfer

the chorizo to a plate, leaving the fat in the skillet; cover the plate to keep warm.

3. Add the poblano and onion to the skillet and season with salt and pepper. Cook, stirring occasionally until golden brown in places and beginning to soften, 7 to 8 minutes. Add a bit more oil if needed during the cooking process. Transfer to a plate and cover.

4. Add 1 teaspoon of oil to the skillet. Add the eggplant slices and cook until tender, about 3 minutes on each side. Transfer to a plate lined with a paper towel to absorb any excess oil.

5. Add the remaining 1 teaspoon oil to the skillet. Crack the eggs into the skillet, season with salt and pepper, and fry until the whites are set and the yolks are still runny, about 3 minutes.

6. While the eggs are cooking, place an eggplant slice on each plate and spread the chipotle crema on the eggplant. Add the chorizo and poblano-onion mix on top of the eggplant. Top with the fried eggs, avocado, and purslane and serve.

Sicilian Breakfast Salad

Serves 4

2 teaspoons balsamic vinegar
¼ cup extra virgin olive oil
¼ teaspoon kosher salt
pinch red pepper flakes
6 cups dandelion greens, cut into 1-inch pieces
¼ cup pomegranate seeds (see Note)
¼ cup sliced almonds, toasted
2 ounces ricotta salata, thinly shaved

1. In a small bowl, whisk together the vinegar and oil until smooth. Season with the salt and red pepper flakes and set aside.

2. In a large bowl, toss the dandelion greens and the pomegranate seeds. Divide evenly among four serving bowls, top with the almonds, cheese, and dressing, and serve.

NOTE ···

To extract pomegranate seeds, you can do what my grand-mother used to do: Halve the fruit, hold each half, cut-side down, over a bowl, and whack it with a wooden spoon. Alternatively, you can do what I do: Press each half on a juicer to remove the seeds and discard the juice (which is too sweet to use).

···

Protein Crêpes with Turkey Sausage

Serves 3

4½ teaspoons grass-fed butter, divided

3 turkey sausage links, cut into ¼-inch-thick pieces

1 small red bell pepper, seeded and chopped

1 small yellow bell pepper, seeded and chopped

2 tablespoons water

1 tablespoon freshly squeezed lemon juice

½ teaspoon ground cinnamon, plus more for garnish

3 tablespoons plus ½ teaspoon stevia, divided

1 scoop vanilla whey protein powder

⅔ cup egg whites

1 tablespoon unsweetened vanilla almond milk

1 tablespoon ground flaxseed

1 tablespoon unsweetened coconut flour

½ cup mascarpone cheese

15 drops SweetLeaf Liquid Stevia Sweet Drops, vanilla crème flavor

1. In a sauté pan, melt 2 teaspoons of the butter over medium heat. Add the sausage, red and yellow bell peppers, water, lemon juice, cinnamon, and 3 tablespoons of the stevia. Sauté until the sausage appears cooked, about 10 minutes. Cover and set aside.

2. Combine the whey protein, egg whites, almond milk, flaxseed, coconut flour, remaining ½ teaspoon stevia, and 1 teaspoon of the butter to a blender or food processor. Blend until a batter forms.

3. Melt ½ teaspoon of the butter in a large sauté pan over medium heat. Pour one-third of the batter into the pan and tilt the pan to

spread a thin layer evenly over the bottom of the pan. When the edges start to slightly brown, carefully flip the crêpe with a spatula. When the other side is cooked, transfer the crêpe to a plate. Repeat with the remaining mixture and butter to make two more crêpes. This step happens quickly, so be careful not to look away.

4. Spread one-third of the sausage mixture onto each crêpe, then fold each lengthwise and then over on itself (like a hot dog bun and then like a hamburger bun).

5. In a small bowl, whisk together the mascarpone and the vanilla crème stevia drops. Top each crepe with one-third of the mixture, garnish with cinnamon, and serve.

Protein Crêpes with Lox and Cream Cheese

Serves 3

1 scoop vanilla whey protein powder
⅔ cup egg whites
1 tablespoon unsweetened vanilla almond milk
1 tablespoon ground flaxseed
1 tablespoon unsweetened coconut flour
½ teaspoon stevia
2½ teaspoons unsalted grass-fed butter, divided
4 ounces lox
½ cup cream cheese
2 scallions, chopped

1. Combine the whey protein, egg whites, almond milk, flaxseed, coconut flour, stevia, and 1 teaspoon of the butter in a blender or food processor. Blend until a batter forms.

2. Melt ½ teaspoon of the butter in a large sauté pan over medium heat. Pour one-third of the batter into the pan and tilt the pan to spread a thin layer evenly over the bottom of the pan. When the edges start to slightly brown, carefully flip the crêpe with a spatula. When the other side is cooked, transfer the crêpe to a plate. Repeat with the remaining mixture to make two more crêpes. This step happens quickly, so be careful not to look away.

3. Spread one-third of the lox and cream cheese onto each crepe, then fold each lengthwise and then over on itself (like a hot dog bun and then like a hamburger bun). Sprinkle with chopped scallions and serve.

Pumpkin Protein Pancakes

Serves 2

2 scoops protein powder
½ cup diced pumpkin
½ teaspoon ground cinnamon (or ¼ teaspoon pumpkin pie spice + ¼ teaspoon ground cinnamon)
2 large egg whites
3 to 5 packets SweetLeaf® stevia
1 teaspoon unsalted grass-fed butter
1 tablespoon coconut flour
macadamia nut oil spray

1. Combine all the ingredients (except the spray) in a blender and blend until smooth.
2. Spray a bit of macadamia nut oil onto a nonstick griddle or large nonstick skillet and place over medium heat. Spoon about ¼ cup of batter per pancake onto the griddle. Turn the pancakes over when the tops are covered with bubbles and the edges look cooked. Cook the other side, then serve.

Rainbow Chard Frittata

Serves 8

2 tablespoons unsalted grass-fed butter, divided
1 small red onion, chopped
1 bunch rainbow Swiss chard (14 ounces), leaves coarsely chopped, stems cut into 1-inch pieces
coarse sea salt and freshly ground black pepper

5 ostrich eggs, at room temperature
1½ cups heavy cream
1 tablespoon Dijon mustard
¼ teaspoon freshly grated nutmeg
½ cup sour cream
3 tablespoons harissa

1. Preheat the oven to 350°F.
2. Melt 1 tablespoon of the butter in a large cast-iron or oven-safe skillet over medium heat. Add the onion and chard leaves and season with salt and pepper. Cook, stirring occasionally, until the chard wilts and becomes tender, about 7 minutes. Transfer to a plate and let cool completely.
3. Meanwhile, blanch the chard stems in a pot of generously salted boiling water until crisp-tender and more vibrant in color, 2 minutes or less. Drain, transfer to another plate, and let cool completely.
4. In a large bowl, whisk together the eggs, cream, and Dijon. Season with salt and pepper.
5. Melt the remaining 1 tablespoon butter in the same skillet over low heat. Remove the skillet from the heat and spread the chard leaf and onion mixture evenly over the bottom of the skillet. Pour the egg mixture over the chard and sprinkle the nutmeg evenly over the top.
6. Bake until the eggs begin to set at the edges, about 20 minutes.
7. Scatter the chard stems evenly over the top of the eggs. Return the skillet to the oven and continue baking until the eggs are set in the center. Depending on your oven, this should be another 10 to 20 minutes.
8. Set the skillet on a wire rack to cool for 15 minutes before cutting the frittata into wedges.
9. Whisk together the sour cream and harissa and dollop on top of each serving. Serve.

NOTE

This is a great recipe that you can make once and then eat for the entire week, for lunch or a quick snack.

Spaghetti Squash, Taleggio, and Okra Frittata

Serves 2

1 spaghetti squash
1 tablespoon macadamia nut oil
1 shallot, diced
1 cup finely diced mustard greens
½ cup thinly sliced okra
¼ cup shredded Taleggio cheese
4 large eggs, whisked

1. Preheat the oven to 300°F. Butter a 9-inch round cake pan.
2. Cut the spaghetti squash in half and discard the seeds. Place half of the squash, cut-side down, on a baking sheet. Bake until fork tender, 20 to 25 minutes. (Reserve the other half of the squash for another meal or double this recipe for friends or to eat later in the week.)
3. Meanwhile, heat the oil in a large saucepan over medium heat. Add the shallot and cook until translucent, about 5 minutes. Add the mustard greens and okra and cook for 4 minutes. Remove from the heat and set aside to cool.
4. When the squash is done, use a fork to remove the threads of squash and place them in a bowl.
5. Add the vegetable mixture and shredded cheese to the squash and stir to combine. Pour in the eggs and stir to combine.
6. Transfer the mixture to the prepared cake pan and spread evenly.
7. Bake for 45 minutes. Let cool on a rack slightly before serving.

Chicken Breakfast Skillet

Serves 1

1 teaspoon macadamia nut oil
1 chicken sausage link, diced
½ cup diced shiitake mushrooms

⅓ cup diced orange bell pepper
½ cup diced cipollini onion
½ teaspoon garlic powder
½ teaspoon smoked paprika
¼ teaspoon cayenne pepper
coarse sea salt and freshly ground black pepper
3 large eggs

1. Preheat the oven to 400°F.
2. Heat the oil in a cast-iron skillet over medium-high heat. Add the sausage and sauté until the fat from the sausage is rendered, about 10 minutes.
3. Add the mushrooms, orange bell pepper, onion, garlic powder, paprika, and cayenne and stir to combine.
4. Make three wells in the mixture, crack an egg into each one, and season with salt and pepper. Transfer the skillet to the oven and bake for 5 to 10 minutes, depending on how you like your yolk. Serve.

Duck Eggs with Brussels Sprouts and Pancetta

Serves 2

3 teaspoons macadamia nut oil, divided
3 ounces pancetta, cut into thin strips
6 ounces Brussels sprouts, trimmed and thinly sliced lengthwise
coarse sea salt and freshly ground black pepper
1 large portobello mushroom cap
2 duck eggs
Dijon mustard, to taste
2 parsley sprigs

1. In a large cast-iron or nonstick skillet, heat 2 teaspoons of the oil over medium-high heat. Add the pancetta and cook, stirring occasionally, until beginning to brown and the fat starts to render, 2 to 3 minutes.
2. Add the Brussels sprouts and season with salt and pepper. Cook, stirring occasionally, until the sprouts are crisp-tender, about 5

minutes. Using a slotted spoon, transfer the sprouts and pancetta to a plate and cover to keep warm.

3. Put the portobello mushroom cap in the skillet and cook each side for about 2 minutes—don't let it get soggy. Cut the mushroom cap in half and place one half on each plate.

4. Wipe down the skillet to remove any liquid from the mushroom and add the remaining 1 teaspoon oil. Reduce the heat to medium and crack the eggs into the skillet. Season with salt and pepper and fry until the whites are set and the yolks are still runny, about 3 minutes.

5. To assemble, spread a little Dijon on the mushrooms, divide the Brussels sprouts and pancetta evenly over the mushrooms, and top each with an egg. Add a sprig of parsley to each plate and serve.

Egg Foo Young with Oysters

Serves 4

2 tablespoons macadamia nut oil, divided
6 medium oysters, shucked
8 ounces bean sprouts, root ends trimmed
1 celery stalk, cut into ½-inch julienne strips
1 scallion, cut into 1½-inch pieces
2 tablespoons tamari
12 duck eggs
1 teaspoon coarse sea salt
2 tablespoons almond flour
2 tablespoons water

1. Heat 1 tablespoon of the oil in a large cast-iron or nonstick skillet over medium-high heat. Add the oysters and stir-fry for 1 minute. Add the bean sprouts, celery, scallion, and tamari and stir-fry for another minute. Transfer the mixture to a large bowl.

2. In another large bowl, lightly whisk the eggs with the salt. Heat the remaining 1 tablespoon oil in the same skillet over medium-high heat and pour in the eggs. Cook without stirring them, lifting the edges occasionally and letting the uncooked portion run under the cooked part.

3. When the eggs are firm but still partly liquid, drain the oyster mixture through a sieve placed over a bowl. Reserve the liquid and spread the oyster mixture over the eggs.

4. Fold half of the egg mixture over the other to make a semi-circular omelet. Cook for 1½ minutes, then lift up the curved side with a spatula and gently flip the omelet onto the other side. Cook for 1½ minutes more. Transfer to a heated platter and cover to keep warm.

5. To make the gravy, pour the reserved oyster-mixture liquid into the same skillet. Heat to boiling over medium heat.

6. In a cup, whisk the almond flour into the water until dissolved, then whisk this into the skillet. Boil for another 1 to 2 minutes until slightly thick and pour over the eggs. Serve.

Shakshuka

Serves 3

3 tablespoons macadamia nut oil
1 large onion, halved lengthwise and thinly sliced crosswise
1 large red bell pepper, seeded and thinly sliced
3 garlic cloves, thinly sliced
2 tablespoons harissa
1 teaspoon ground cumin
1 teaspoon sweet paprika
⅛ teaspoon cayenne pepper, or to taste
3 plum tomatoes, coarsely chopped, with their juices
¾ teaspoon coarse sea salt, or more if needed
¼ teaspoon freshly ground black pepper, or more if needed
5 ounces feta cheese, crumbled (about 1¼ cups)
6 large eggs
chopped fresh cilantro, for garnish

1. Preheat the oven to 375°F.
2. Heat the oil in a large oven-safe skillet over medium-low heat. Add the onion and bell pepper. Cook gently until very soft, about 20 minutes. Add the garlic and cook until tender, 1 to 2 minutes. Stir in the harissa, cumin, paprika, and cayenne and cook for 1

minute. Pour in the tomatoes and their juices and add the salt and black pepper. Simmer until the tomatoes have thickened, about 10 minutes. Stir in the crumbled feta.

3. Make 6 little wells in the mixture and gently crack an egg into each well. Season with salt and pepper.

4. Transfer the skillet to the oven and bake until the eggs are just set, 7 to 10 minutes.

5. Let the shakshuka sit for 3 minutes, then sprinkle with the cilantro and serve.

NOTE
This classic Middle Eastern dish can be served for dinner, although traditionally it is a breakfast dish.

Japanese Eggs with Radish

Serves 4

⅔ cup white vinegar
⅔ cup water
½ teaspoon coarse sea salt
4 hard-boiled eggs, peeled
2 garlic cloves, peeled and smashed
1 teaspoon whole black peppercorns
8 radishes, thinly sliced
1 avocado, peeled and pitted
juice of ½ lemon
¼ teaspoon chili powder
¼ cup chopped fresh cilantro
3 chives, diced
freshly ground black pepper

1. In a medium saucepan, bring the vinegar, water, and salt to a boil over medium heat. Simmer for 1 minute, then set aside to cool.

2. Place the eggs, garlic, and peppercorns in a clean jar and pour in the cooled vinegar mixture. Seal the jar and chill in the fridge for at least 1 day to pickle.

3. To serve, divide the radish slices among four plates.
4. In a medium bowl, mash together the avocado, lemon juice, and chili powder with a fork until chunky. Spread this mixture over the radishes.
5. Slice the pickled eggs and divide among the plates. Garnish with cilantro, chives, and black pepper and serve.

Breakfast Tartlets

Makes 12

1½ cups ricotta
2 tablespoons macadamia nut oil
½ garlic clove, minced
grated zest of ½ lemon
½ teaspoon Tabasco
1 teaspoon coarse sea salt, plus more for sprinkling
2 large cucumbers, peeled
3 tablespoons unsalted grass-fed butter, divided
5 large eggs, whisked
freshly ground white pepper
2 tablespoons heavy cream
6 prosciutto slices, torn in half lengthwise
½ bunch fresh watercress
freshly ground black pepper

1. In a bowl, whisk together the ricotta, oil, garlic, lemon zest, Tabasco, and salt until the oil is emulsified and the ricotta is light and smooth. Set aside.
2. Using a mandoline, slice the cucumber into almost transparent slices. Stack the slices into 12 rounds.
3. In a medium sauté pan, melt 1 tablespoon of the butter over medium heat. Add the eggs and cook, stirring constantly. Season with salt and white pepper.
4. When the eggs are half cooked but still very runny, remove the pan from the heat and stir in the remaining 2 tablespoons butter and the cream. The eggs should look like oatmeal.

5. Spread 1 tablespoon of the ricotta mixture onto each stack
    of cucumber slices. Top with a spoonful of egg and a strip of
    prosciutto. Garnish with watercress and black pepper and serve.

    NOTE
    You can serve two of these for breakfast or three for lunch.

Smoked Mackerel Cakes

Serves 6

macadamia nut oil spray
1 tablespoon macadamia nut oil
1 onion, diced
8 ounces cremini mushrooms, chopped
1 orange bell pepper, seeded and chopped
3 cups chopped spinach
1 cup ricotta cheese
8 duck eggs
8 ounces skinless smoked mackerel, roughly chopped
3 tablespoons chopped fresh dill
3 tablespoons prepared horseradish
1 tablespoon Dijon mustard
½ teaspoon freshly ground white pepper

1. Preheat the oven to 375°F. Coat a 12-cup muffin tin with
    macadamia nut oil spray.
2. Heat the oil in a cast-iron skillet over medium heat. Add the
    onion, mushrooms, and bell pepper. Sauté until softened, about 6
    minutes. Stir in the spinach until slightly wilted and remove the
    pan from the heat.
3. In a large bowl, whisk together the ricotta and eggs. Stir in the
    cooked vegetables, mackerel, dill, horseradish, mustard, and pepper.
4. Divide the mixture among the muffin cups. Bake until the eggs are
    set, about 20 minutes.
5. Let cool for 5 minutes before unmolding. Serve.

Parmesan Crisps Topped with Bacon, Egg, Pistachios, and Parsley

Serves 2

½ cup grated Parmesan cheese
4 bacon slices
2 large eggs
20 pistachios
½ cup fresh parsley

1. Preheat the oven to 375°F.
2. Divide the Parmesan into two equal mounds on a baking sheet and gently flatten each mound into a 4½- to 5-inch circle. Bake until golden and bubbly, 8 to 10 minutes. Let cool until firm, about 5 minutes.
3. In a medium sauté pan, cook the bacon to your desired crispness. Transfer to a paper towel to drain. When cool, crumble it into bits.
4. Crack the eggs into the same pan and cook until the white is firm but not done, about 3 minutes, then carefully flip over. Cook until done, about 3 additional minutes.
5. In a mini food processor, pulse the pistachios and parsley until completely combined.
6. Place one Parmesan circle on each plate. On each circle, spread some pistachio and parsley mixture and top with a fried egg. Sprinkle with the bacon bits and serve.

Portobello Mushroom Topped with Scrambled Eggs

Serves 2

⅓ cup sour cream
1 tablespoon macadamia nut oil, plus more for brushing
1 teaspoon minced chipotles in adobo
1 garlic clove, minced

2 large portobello mushroom caps
coarse sea salt
8 quail eggs
freshly ground black pepper
macadamia nut oil spray
1 cup arugula

1. Preheat the broiler.
2. In a bowl, whisk together the sour cream, oil, chipotle, and garlic and set aside.
3. Place the portobello caps, cap-side up, on a baking sheet. Brush the tops lightly with oil and season with salt. Broil until tender, about 5 minutes.
4. In another bowl, whisk the eggs and season with salt and pepper. Coat a large skillet with macadamia nut oil spray and pour in the eggs. Cook over medium-low heat, stirring frequently, until creamy curds form, about 3 to 4 minutes. Remove the skillet from the heat while the eggs are still runny.
5. Place the portobellos, cap-side up, on serving plates and top each with eggs, sour cream sauce, and arugula. Serve.

Avocado Smoothie

Serves 1 or 2

4 cups spinach
1 Lebanese cucumber, peeled
2 limes, peeled
1 medium-large avocado, peeled and pitted
½ cup unsweetened almond milk
stevia, to taste
1 cup ice

Combine all the ingredients in a high-speed blender and puree until smooth. Serve immediately.

Soups

Garlic Soup with Mascarpone and Chives

Serves 4

10 heads garlic, cloves separated and peeled
1 quart chicken or vegetable broth
coarse sea salt and freshly ground black pepper
½ cup heavy cream
½ cup mascarpone
4 chives, finely chopped

1. Put the peeled garlic cloves in a large stockpot and add enough water to cover them by 2 inches. Bring the water to a boil over high heat and then drain the water. Repeat this step twice and then return the garlic to the pot.
2. Add the broth and season with salt and pepper. Bring the broth to a boil over high heat.
3. Decrease the heat and simmer until the garlic is tender, about 15 minutes. Remove the pot from the heat and allow the soup to cool.
4. Transfer the soup to a blender and puree until smooth.
5. Return the soup to the pot and whisk in the cream. Bring to a simmer over low heat.
6. Divide the soup among four bowls, top with the mascarpone, and sprinkle with chives. Serve.

Vegetable Soup

Serves 2

1 tablespoon macadamia nut oil
¼ white onion, finely chopped
2 large scallions, finely chopped
3 garlic cloves, minced
2 celery stalks, finely chopped
2 medium carrots, peeled and finely chopped
2 cups vegetable broth
1 cup broccoli florets

¼ cup chopped fresh purslane
1 bay leaf
½ teaspoon ground ginger
1 teaspoon coarse sea salt
2 cups baby spinach
2 large kale leaves, coarsely chopped
1 tablespoon tamari
1 teaspoon freshly squeezed lemon juice
2 teaspoons extra virgin olive oil, for drizzling

1. In a medium stockpot, heat the oil over medium-high heat. Add the onion, scallions, garlic, celery, and carrot and sauté until soft, about 5 minutes.
2. Add the broth, broccoli, purslane, bay leaf, ginger, and salt and cook until the broccoli is soft, about 5 minutes.
3. Add the spinach and kale and stir well.
4. Add the tamari and lemon juice and adjust the seasoning to taste.
5. Divide the soup between two bowls, drizzle 1 teaspoon olive oil over each, and serve.

Creole Gumbo

Serves 4

4 ounces okra, cut into ½-inch-thick rounds
2 tablespoons white vinegar
½ teaspoon kosher salt
3 tablespoons macadamia nut oil, divided
1 onion, chopped
2 celery stalks, chopped
1 green bell pepper, seeded and chopped
3 garlic cloves, minced
1 bay leaf, crumbled
1 teaspoon dried thyme
½ teaspoon dried oregano
¼ teaspoon cayenne pepper
5 cups chicken broth

1 pound Italian sausage, cut into ½-inch-thick slices
18 medium shrimp, peeled and deveined
18 oysters, shucked

1. In a medium bowl, toss together the okra, vinegar, and salt. Set aside.
2. In a large stockpot, heat 2 tablespoons of the oil over medium heat. Add the onion, celery, bell pepper, and garlic and sauté until well wilted but not browned, 10 to 12 minutes.
3. Stir in the bay leaf, thyme, oregano, and cayenne. Add the broth and bring to a boil. Decrease the heat and simmer for 30 minutes.
4. While the broth simmers, heat the remaining 1 tablespoon oil in a large sauté pan over medium-high heat. Cook the sausage, browning it for about 4 minutes on each side. Transfer the sausage to the soup pot.
5. Rinse the okra and transfer it to the soup pot. Let the soup simmer for 15 minutes. Add the shrimp and oysters, cover the pot, and remove from the heat.
6. Let the soup stand until the shrimp are barely pink and the oysters are slightly plump, about 6 minutes. Serve.

Creamy Avocado-Broccoflower Soup

Serves 4

2 cups vegetable broth
1 yellow onion, chopped
3 cups broccoflower florets
1 small avocado, peeled and pitted
1 green bell pepper, cored and seeded
1 red bell pepper, cored and seeded
1 celery stalk, coarsely chopped
½ teaspoon ground turmeric
½ teaspoon ground cumin
½ teaspoon dried basil
coarse sea salt

1. In a medium stockpot, heat the vegetable broth over medium heat but do not boil.

2.   Add the onion and broccoflower and warm for several minutes.
3.   Remove the pot from the heat and transfer the soup to a blender. Add the avocado, bell peppers, and celery and puree until the soup is creamy (add more water or broth if desired).
4.   Add the turmeric, cumin, and basil and season with salt. Reblend and serve warm.

Swiss Cauliflower-Emmentaler Soup

Serves 2

2 cups vegetable broth
2 cups cauliflower florets
pinch ground nutmeg
pinch cayenne pepper
coarse sea salt and freshly ground black pepper
3 ounces Emmentaler cheese, cubed
2 tablespoons minced chives
1 tablespoon pumpkin seeds, toasted

1.   In a medium stockpot, heat the vegetable broth over medium heat but do not boil. Add the cauliflower and cook until tender, 5 to 7 minutes.
2.   Transfer the mixture to a blender and puree. Add the nutmeg and cayenne and season with salt and black pepper.
3.   Pour the soup into a large serving bowl. Add the cheese and chives and stir until the soup is smooth.
4.   Garnish with the toasted pumpkin seeds and serve.

Parsley Gazpacho

Serves 4

2 tablespoons macadamia nut oil
2 small red onions, roughly chopped
2 garlic cloves, minced
2 cups minced fresh parsley

2 avocados, peeled and pitted
1 medium cucumber, sliced
4 cups vegetable broth
juice of 2 limes
1½ teaspoons paprika
1 teaspoon dried oregano
½ teaspoon cayenne pepper
coarse sea salt and freshly ground black pepper
4 chives, minced
4 dill sprigs

1. In a medium sauté pan, heat the oil over medium heat. Add the onions and garlic and sauté until translucent, about 5 minutes. Remove the pan from the heat and set aside to cool.
2. In a blender, combine the parsley, avocados, cucumber, broth, lime juice, onion-garlic mixture, paprika, oregano, and cayenne. Puree until smooth (you may need to do this in two batches). Add some water if desired, and season with salt and black pepper.
3. Blend again, cover, and chill in the fridge for at least 1½ hours.
4. To serve, ladle into four soup bowls and garnish each serving with some chives and a sprig of dill.

Turkey Chili

Serves 8

1 cup macadamia nut oil
1 large onion, diced
2 large garlic cloves, minced
1 medium jalapeño, seeded and minced
2 pounds ground turkey breast
1 teaspoon coarse sea salt
1½ cups water
4 plum tomatoes, coarsely chopped, with their juices
2 tablespoons dried oregano
2 tablespoons ground cumin
2 tablespoons ground turmeric

1 tablespoon cayenne pepper
1 teaspoon smoked paprika
½ teaspoon black pepper
2 avocados, peeled and pitted
1 bunch cilantro, chopped
1 scallion, chopped

1. Heat the oil in a large, heavy-bottomed pan over medium heat. Add the onion and cook until translucent, 3 to 5 minutes. Add the garlic and jalapeño and cook for another minute.
2. Stir in the ground turkey and salt and cook, breaking up the pieces with a spoon, until no longer pink, about 5 minutes.
3. Add the water, tomatoes and their juices, oregano, cumin, turmeric, cayenne, smoked paprika, and black pepper. Cook for 30 minutes at a gentle simmer, stirring occasionally.
4. Puree the avocados in a food processor or blender until smooth and creamy. Stir the avocado mixture into the soup and simmer for an additional 30 minutes.
5. To serve, ladle the chili into soup bowls and garnish with cilantro and scallion.

Almond Soup with Lump Crab

Serves 10 to 12

1 tablespoon macadamia nut oil
1 medium carrot, peeled and coarsely chopped (½ cup)
1 medium onion, finely diced
coarse sea salt
4 cups unsalted roasted almonds (or any nut you like)
8 cups chicken broth
3 cups water
3 tablespoons freshly squeezed lemon juice
freshly ground black pepper
2 pounds jumbo lump crab
red pepper flakes, for garnish
avocado oil, for drizzling

1. Heat the oil in a large pot over medium heat. Add the carrot and onion and season with salt. Cook, stirring occasionally until the vegetables are soft, about 5 minutes.
2. Add the almonds, broth, and water and bring to a boil. Decrease the heat and simmer until the nuts are tender, 1¼ to 1½ hours.
3. For this step, you will need to work in batches: Pour enough soup to fill your blender halfway and puree until smooth, about 1 minute. Strain each batch through a fine-mesh sieve set over a separate pot, pressing on the solids to squeeze out as much liquid as possible. Discard the solids in the sieve. Repeat this step until all the soup has been pureed and sieved.
4. Set the pot over low heat and stir in the lemon juice. Season with salt and pepper and ladle into soup bowls.
5. Drop equal portions of the lump crab into each soup bowl, sprinkle with red pepper flakes, and add a drizzle of avocado oil. Serve.

Fish Broth

Makes 1 quart

1 tablespoon macadamia nut oil
2 pounds fish bones
2 large shallots, sliced
6 parsley stems
2 teaspoons fine sea salt
½ teaspoon white peppercorns
½ teaspoon fennel seeds
½ teaspoon fenugreek seeds
½ teaspoon coriander seeds
1 cup dry white wine
1 quart water

1. Heat the oil in a large saucepan over medium heat. Add the fish bones, shallots, parsley, and seasonings. Cook, stirring, until fragrant, about 4 minutes.

2. Add the wine and reduce by half. Add the water and gently simmer for 30 minutes.

3. Strain the fish broth through a sieve and discard the solids.

NOTE
You can use this same recipe to make many different bone broths (such as poultry or beef).

Sea Bass Stew

Serves 6

FOR THE AIOLI
2 large garlic cloves, peeled
2 large egg yolks
¼ cup Fish Broth (page 186)
1½ teaspoons Dijon mustard
¾ teaspoon coarse sea salt
⅛ teaspoon cayenne pepper
½ cup macadamia nut oil
¼ cup extra virgin olive oil

FOR THE STEW
1 quart Fish Broth (page 186)
3 small carrots, peeled and cut into ¼-inch-thick pieces
8 ounces white button mushrooms, quartered
1 leek, light green and white parts only, cut into ¼-inch pieces
1 small fennel bulb, trimmed and cut into ¼-inch pieces
3 whole sea bass (about 3 pounds altogether), skinned, deboned, and filleted into 6 pieces (see Note)
sea salt and freshly ground white pepper
cayenne pepper
juice of 1 lemon
¼ cup fresh parsley leaves, for garnish

1. To make the aioli, combine the garlic cloves, egg yolks, fish broth, mustard, salt, and cayenne in a blender and puree until smooth.

While the blender is running, add the oils in a slow, steady stream. The sauce should emulsify into a thick consistency similar to mayonnaise. Set aside.

2. To make the stew, in a medium saucepot, heat the fish broth to a simmer over medium heat.

3. Add the carrots, mushrooms, leek, and fennel, cover, and gently simmer until the vegetables are tender, about 8 minutes.

4. Meanwhile, cut the fillets into 1-inch pieces and season with salt, white pepper, and cayenne.

5. Add the fish to the soup, cover, and cook until translucent, 3 to 4 minutes. With a slotted spoon, scoop the fish and vegetables from the broth and divide among six warm soup bowls; cover each with plastic wrap.

6. Transfer the broth to the blender with the aioli and puree until smooth. Add the lemon juice and adjust the seasonings to taste. To serve, ladle the broth mixture into the soup bowls and sprinkle with the parsley leaves.

NOTE

Have your fishmonger prepare the sea bass for you but retain the bones, which you can use to make Fish Broth (page 186).

Kamut, Lentil, and Chickpea Soup

Serves 6

¾ cup kamut berries, rinsed

2 cups boiling water

2 tablespoons macadamia nut oil

2 cups finely chopped onion

1 cup finely chopped carrot

½ cup thinly sliced celery

¾ cup chopped fresh parsley

1 tablespoon chopped fresh tarragon

2 teaspoons chopped fresh thyme

2 garlic cloves, minced
2 quarts chicken broth
2 bay leaves
⅓ cup dried lentils
¼ teaspoon freshly ground black pepper
1 (15-ounce) can chickpeas (garbanzo beans), rinsed and drained
2 teaspoons chopped celery leaves

1. Put the kamut in a small bowl. Carefully pour the boiling water over it. Let stand for 30 minutes, then drain.
2. Heat the oil in a large stockpot over medium heat. Add the onion, carrot, celery, parsley, tarragon, and thyme and cook for 10 minutes, stirring occasionally. Add the garlic and cook for 2 minutes, stirring often.
3. Add the kamut, broth, and bay leaves and bring to a boil. Cover, decrease the heat, and simmer for 30 minutes. Add the lentils and black pepper and cook until the lentils are tender, about 20 minutes.
4. Discard the bay leaves. Add the chickpeas and simmer for 2 minutes. To serve, ladle the soup into bowls and garnish with the celery leaves.

Salads

Bitter Greens, Grapefruit, and Avocado Salad

Serves 6

1 pink grapefruit
2 teaspoons champagne vinegar
¼ cup sour cream
1 teaspoon Dijon mustard
¼ teaspoon kosher salt
¼ teaspoon freshly ground white pepper
¼ cup extra virgin olive oil
2 heads Belgian endive (red or white), leaves coarsely chopped (4 cups)
2 heads frisée, leaves torn into bite-size pieces (2 cups)
½ head escarole, leaves coarsely chopped (4 cups)
1 cup fresh mint leaves
1 avocado, peeled, pitted, and thinly sliced
flaxseed, for garnish

1. Remove the peel and pith from the grapefruit. Working over a bowl to catch the juice, carefully cut between the membranes to remove each whole segment. Set aside.
2. In a small bowl, whisk together 2 tablespoons of the grapefruit juice, vinegar, sour cream, Dijon, salt, and white pepper. Slowly drizzle in the olive oil and whisk until combined.
3. In a large bowl, toss together the endive, frisée, escarole, and mint. Divide the salad evenly among six plates.
4. Top with the grapefruit and avocado slices. To serve, drizzle with the vinaigrette and sprinkle with flaxseed.

NOTE
Salad dressings can usually be stored in the refrigerator for 2 or 3 days, so you can make it ahead of time or make extra—simply whisk it until smooth before serving.

Kohlrabi Salad with Vegetable Dressing

Serves 2

3 tablespoons extra virgin olive oil
juice of ½ lemon
coarse sea salt and freshly ground black pepper
¼ cup fresh radish sprouts
1 spring onion or shallot, minced
3 green kohlrabi, peeled and very thinly sliced

1. In a small bowl, whisk together the oil and lemon juice and season with salt and pepper. Add the sprouts and then mix in the onion.
2. Divide the kohlrabi slices between two plates and cover each with the dressing. Serve.

Raw Kale and Hemp Seed Salad

Serves 4

1 bunch Lacinato kale, stems removed and leaves chopped
1 avocado, peeled, pitted, and cubed
1 cup cherry tomatoes, halved
2 tablespoons hemp seeds
20 pistachios, crushed
2 tablespoons extra virgin olive oil
2 tablespoons champagne vinegar
coarse sea salt and freshly ground black pepper

1. Combine the kale, avocado, cherry tomatoes, hemp seeds, and pistachios in a large bowl. Drizzle with the oil and vinegar and season with salt and pepper. Toss thoroughly, until all the leaves are coated with dressing, seeds, and nuts.
2. Divide among four salad plates and serve.

Asian Vegetable Salad

Serves 4 to 6

1 large bunch cilantro, thick stems removed and remaining
sprigs cut into 3-inch lengths (about 5 cups loosely packed)
1 cucumber, seeded and slivered
1 jalapeño or other fresh chile, stemmed, seeded, and slivered
2 scallions, minced
2 teaspoons macadamia nut oil
¼ teaspoon coarse sea salt
sesame oil, to taste
white vinegar, to taste

1. In a large bowl, combine the cilantro, cucumber, jalapeño, and
    scallions. Add the macadamia nut oil and salt and toss lightly.
2. Add a few drops of sesame oil and vinegar and more salt to taste;
    toss again. Serve.

Broccoli and Bacon Salad

Serves 4

2 pounds broccoli florets
10 bacon slices, crisply cooked and crumbled
½ cup chopped red onion
½ cup cashews
½ cup sliced water chestnuts
1 cup lime mayonnaise (page 213) or plain mayonnaise
2 tablespoons white wine vinegar

1. In a large bowl, toss together the broccoli, bacon, onion, cashews,
    and water chestnuts.
2. In a small bowl, whisk together the mayonnaise and vinegar until
    smooth; pour over the salad and toss to coat.
3. Cover the bowl with plastic wrap and refrigerate until the dressing
    sets, at least 4 hours. Serve.

Tuscan Salad with Arctic Char

Serves 2

3 red bell peppers
2 yellow bell peppers
1 cup extra virgin olive oil
¾ cup red wine vinegar
1 teaspoon coarse sea salt
2 tablespoons macadamia nut oil
1 cup asparagus tips
2 (6-ounce) arctic char fillets
kosher salt and freshly ground black pepper
½ lemon
4 cups arugula
1 ounce mozzarella, cubed

1. Preheat the broiler and set the oven rack about 6 inches from the heat source. Line a baking sheet with aluminum foil.
2. Cut the red and yellow peppers in half from top to bottom. Remove the stems, seeds, and ribs, then place the peppers, cut-side down, on the prepared baking sheet.
3. Broil until the skin of the peppers has blackened and blistered, about 5 minutes. Place the blackened peppers in a bowl and cover tightly with plastic wrap. Allow the peppers to steam as they cool, about 20 minutes.
4. Once cool, remove the skins and discard. Transfer two of the roasted red peppers (four halves) to a blender or food processor. Add the olive oil, red wine vinegar, and sea salt and process until smooth; set aside. Thinly slice the remaining roasted red and yellow peppers and set aside.
5. Heat the macadamia nut oil in a grill pan or skillet over medium-high heat. Add the asparagus tips and sauté until they are bright green and crisp-tender, about 2 minutes. Remove and set aside.
6. Season the arctic char fillets with kosher salt and black pepper. Place the fillets in the grill pan or skillet, skin-side up, and cook

until lightly browned, 3 to 4 minutes. Flip the fillets and continue to cook until the fish flakes easily with a fork, 3 to 4 minutes more. Squeeze the lemon juice over the fish and remove from the heat.

7. Meanwhile, toss together the arugula, mozzarella, and red and yellow pepper slices in a large bowl. Toss with 2 tablespoons of the red pepper dressing (reserve the remaining dressing in a covered container in the refrigerator for up to 3 days).

8. Divide the salad between two plates and top each with an arctic char fillet. Serve.

Kale Caesar Salad

Serves 4

FOR THE CAESAR DRESSING

1 ounce anchovy fillets
1 garlic clove, peeled
2 tablespoons red wine vinegar
1 tablespoon white wine vinegar
1 tablespoon freshly squeezed lemon juice
1 teaspoon Dijon mustard
2 dashes Tabasco
2 large egg yolks
1 cup extra virgin olive oil
¼ cup macadamia nut oil
1 cup grated Parmesan cheese
2 tablespoons water

FOR THE SALAD

1 pound Tuscan kale, thinly sliced
1 lemon, cut into ¼-inch-thick slices
coarse sea salt and freshly ground black pepper
¼ cup capers
¼ cup sunflower seeds, toasted
½ cup grated Parmesan cheese

1. To make the dressing, combine the anchovies, garlic, vinegars, lemon juice, mustard, Tabasco, and egg yolks in a blender and puree until smooth. Slowly add the oils, Parmesan, and water and continue to blend until smooth.
2. To make the salad, toss together the kale, lemon slices, and ½ cup of the dressing in a large bowl (reserve the remaining dressing in a covered container in the refrigerator for up to 3 days). Season with salt and pepper to taste.
3. Divide the salad among four bowls and top each with an equal portion of capers, sunflower seeds, and Parmesan. Serve.

Spinach Salad with Pattypan Squash

Serves 4

8 pattypan squash
5 tablespoons macadamia nut oil, divided
1¼ teaspoons coarse sea salt, divided
¼ teaspoon freshly ground black pepper
8 ounces spinach
2 tablespoons freshly squeezed lemon juice
½ teaspoon Dijon mustard
½ teaspoon chia seeds
⅔ cup toasted almonds

1. Preheat the oven to 450°F.
2. Trim the woody ends of the squash and halve each squash crosswise. Scoop out the seeds, leaving a ½-inch-thick shell. Brush the cut sides of the squash shells with 1 tablespoon of the oil and season with ½ teaspoon of the salt and the black pepper. Arrange the squash, cut-side down, on a baking sheet and roast until the squash is tender and the flesh side is browned, about 15 minutes.
3. Transfer the cooked squash to a large bowl, along with the spinach.
4. Combine the remaining 4 tablespoons oil, lemon juice, mustard, chia seeds, and the remaining ¾ teaspoon salt in a jar and shake vigorously, or whisk everything in a small bowl until emulsified.

5. Toss the dressing with the squash and spinach and top with the almonds. Serve.

Chopped Spinach Cobb Salad

Serves 2

FOR THE BLUE CHEESE DRESSING

1 cup mayonnaise
½ cup crumbled blue cheese, divided
½ cup heavy cream
2 tablespoons sour cream
1 tablespoon freshly squeezed lemon juice
1 teaspoon prepared white horseradish
½ teaspoon kosher salt
freshly ground black pepper

FOR THE SALAD

4 cups baby spinach, chopped
6 ounces grilled turkey breast, chopped
2 bacon slices, cooked and crumbled
2 hard-boiled eggs, chopped
2 tablespoons crumbled blue cheese
4 black olives, pitted and chopped

1. To make the dressing, in a medium bowl whisk together the mayonnaise, ¼ cup of the blue cheese, heavy cream, sour cream, lemon juice, horseradish, and salt until smooth. Gently stir in the remaining ¼ cup blue cheese and season with black pepper.
2. To make the salad, combine all the ingredients in a large bowl. Add ¼ cup of the dressing and toss well. (Reserve the remaining dressing in a covered container in the refrigerator for up to 3 days.) Divide between two salad bowls and serve.

NOTE
You can use the leftover blue cheese dressing for another salad later in the week, such as the Astoria Greek Salad (page 198).

Fennel and Avocado Salad

Serves 2

1 fennel bulb
1 avocado, peeled, pitted, and halved
2 teaspoons freshly squeezed lemon juice
¼ cup thinly sliced red onion, rinsed and patted dry
3 tablespoons red wine vinegar
1 tablespoon extra virgin olive oil
½ teaspoon fine sea salt, or more to taste
freshly ground black pepper, to taste
½ teaspoon red pepper flakes
½ teaspoon dried dill

1. Trim and discard the stems and tough outer skin of the fennel. Cut the fennel lengthwise into quarters, then crosswise into thin slices. (There should be about 1½ cups.) Put in a medium bowl.
2. Cut the avocado halves lengthwise into quarters, then crosswise into ½-inch pieces. (There should be about 4 cups.) Add the avocado to the fennel.
3. Add the lemon juice and toss to blend. Add the onion slices.
4. Add the vinegar, oil, salt, black pepper, red pepper flakes, and dill. Toss and serve.

The Astoria Greek Salad

Serves 2

4 cups chopped romaine lettuce
2 cups chopped purslane
1 red bell pepper, seeded and chopped
1 green bell pepper, seeded and chopped
½ medium cucumber, peeled and diced
2 celery stalks, diced
2 (6-ounce) grilled chicken breasts, chopped
6 Kalamata olives, pitted and halved

2 tablespoons blue cheese dressing (page 197)
3 tablespoons feta cheese

1. In a medium bowl, toss together the lettuce, purslane, bell peppers, cucumber, celery, chicken, and olives.
2. Add the dressing and toss again. Top with the feta cheese and serve.

Avocado Salad with Alfalfa Sprouts

Serves 4

2 avocados, peeled, pitted, and diced
2 tablespoons freshly squeezed lime juice, divided
5 to 6 ounces alfalfa sprouts
1 garlic clove, minced
¼ cup cold pressed extra virgin olive oil
4 fresh basil leaves, minced
coarse sea salt and freshly ground black pepper

1. Put the avocados in a bowl and sprinkle with ½ tablespoon of the lime juice. Add the alfalfa sprouts.
2. In another bowl, mix the garlic with the remaining 1½ tablespoons lime juice, olive oil, and basil. Season with salt and pepper.
3. Stir the dressing into the avocado mixture and serve.

Frisée and Radicchio Salad with Mustard Vinaigrette

Serves 4

6 ounces frisée, stems trimmed and leaves torn into pieces
½ small head radicchio, cored and thinly sliced
1 tablespoon fresh tarragon leaves
1 teaspoon Dijon mustard
1½ teaspoons freshly squeezed lemon juice
3 tablespoons extra virgin olive oil
coarse sea salt and freshly ground black pepper

1. In a large bowl, toss together the frisée, radicchio, and tarragon leaves.
2. In a small bowl, whisk together the mustard and lemon juice. Slowly whisk in the oil until an emulsion forms. Season with salt and pepper and whisk for an additional minute.
3. Drizzle the dressing over the salad and toss before serving.

NOTE
This salad goes well with Grilled Cashew Chicken (page 211).

Spelt Salad with Beans and Artichokes

Serves 6

1¼ cups uncooked spelt, rinsed and drained
2½ cups water
1 (15-ounce) can navy beans, rinsed and drained
1 (14-ounce) can artichoke hearts, drained and chopped
¼ cup minced red onion
⅓ cup chopped fresh mint
⅓ cup chopped fresh parsley
3 tablespoons freshly squeezed lemon juice
2 tablespoons macadamia nut oil
¼ teaspoon coarse sea salt
⅛ teaspoon freshly ground black pepper

1. In a medium saucepan, combine the spelt and water and bring to a boil. Cover, decrease the heat, and simmer until the spelt is tender and the liquid is absorbed, about 30 minutes.
2. Combine the cooked spelt and the remaining ingredients in a large bowl and stir well to combine. Cover and chill in the refrigerator until completely cooled, about 2 hours. Serve.

NOTE
This salad can be stored in an airtight container in the refrigerator for several days and eaten as a meal or a snack.

Quinoa Salad

Serves 8

3 quarts water
1½ cups quinoa, rinsed
5 pickling cucumbers, peeled, trimmed, and cut into ¼-inch dice
1 small red onion, cut into ¼-inch dice
1 large tomato, cored, seeded, and diced
1 bunch parsley, stems discarded and leaves chopped
2 bunches mint, stems discarded and leaves chopped
½ cup macadamia nut oil
¼ cup champagne vinegar
juice of 1 lemon
1½ teaspoons coarse sea salt
¾ teaspoon freshly ground black pepper
4 heads endive, trimmed and separated into individual spears
1 avocado, peeled, pitted, and diced, for garnish

1. In a large saucepan, bring the water to a boil over medium heat. Add the quinoa, stir once, and return to a boil. Cook, uncovered, for 12 minutes. Strain the quinoa and rinse well under cold water, shaking the colander well to remove all moisture.
2. Transfer the quinoa to a large bowl. Add the cucumbers, onion, tomato, parsley, mint, oil, vinegar, lemon juice, and salt and pepper and toss well.
3. To serve, spoon the quinoa mixture onto endive spears and top with avocado.

Burgers, Sandwiches, and Melts

My Favorite Burger

Serves 4

1 tablespoon macadamia nut oil, divided
4 medium portobello mushroom caps
1 pound ground beef
1 teaspoon coarse sea salt
1 teaspoon freshly ground black pepper
1 teaspoon ground turmeric
2 cups arugula
2 tablespoons macadamia nut oil
1 large onion, sliced
1 tablespoon lime mayonnaise (page 213) or regular mayonnaise
1 large dill pickle, cut into ¼-inch-thick slices
4 bacon slices, cooked
4 slices horseradish Cheddar cheese

1. Preheat the broiler. Heat an outdoor grill or stovetop grill pan over high heat.
2. Drizzle ½ tablespoon of the oil onto a small baking sheet and place the mushrooms, cap-side down, on the baking sheet. Drizzle the mushrooms with the remaining ½ tablespoon oil and broil for 5 minutes. Turn the caps over and broil for another 5 minutes. Remove from the oven, return the mushrooms to cap-side down, and leave on the baking sheet. Leave the broiler on.
3. Meanwhile, combine the beef, salt, pepper, and turmeric in a bowl and gently mix. Form into four patties. Be careful not to overwork the meat or pack the patties too tightly.
4. Grill the burgers for 2 to 3 minutes on each side. They should be nicely charred but not burnt, medium-rare to medium inside.
5. While the patties are cooking, divide the arugula among the mushroom caps.
6. In a separate small skillet, heat the 2 tablespoons oil over medium-high heat. Add the onion and cook, stirring constantly, until

golden brown, about 10 minutes. Remove from the skillet and drain on a paper towel.

7. Place the cooked burgers on top of the arugula. Spread some mayonnaise on each burger and top with pickles, bacon, caramelized onions, and a slice of cheese.

8. Return the baking sheet to the oven and broil until the cheese melts, about 1 minute. Serve.

Bacon and Blue Cheese Stuffed Burger

Serves 1

6 ounces ground beef
½ teaspoon ground turmeric
¼ teaspoon ground cumin
coarse sea salt and freshly ground black pepper, to taste
2 ounces blue cheese
2 bacon slices, cooked and crumbled
2 tablespoons macadamia nut oil
1 small onion, chopped
2 Napa cabbage leaves

1. In a small bowl, mix the beef, turmeric, cumin, salt and pepper, blue cheese, and bacon. Form into a patty. Be careful not to overwork the meat or pack the patty too tightly. Set aside.

2. In a small skillet, heat the oil over medium-high heat. Add the onion and cook, stirring constantly, until golden brown, about 10 minutes. Remove from the skillet and drain on a paper towel.

3. In the same skillet, cook the burger to the desired temperature, 3 to 5 minutes on each side for medium-rare (which I recommend for this burger so the cheese doesn't fall out).

4. Place the cabbage leaves on a plate. Put the burger on top and then the caramelized onions. Serve.

Chicken Cordon Bleu Wedge Burger

Serves 1

4 ounces ground chicken breast
¼ teaspoon Old Bay Seasoning
1 tablespoon macadamia nut oil
1 slice deli ham
1 slice Swiss cheese
½ head romaine lettuce
2 tablespoons blue cheese dressing (page 197), optional

1. Preheat a stovetop grill pan over high heat.
2. In a small bowl, mix the ground chicken with the Old Bay. Form into a patty.
3. Add the oil to the grill pan. Cook the patty for about 3 minutes on each side. During the last minute of cooking, top the patty with the ham and cheese.
4. Spread out the romaine leaves on a plate. Place the burger on top. Drizzle with blue cheese dressing, if desired, and serve.

Taco Burger Wrap

Serves 1

8 ounces ground beef
½ teaspoon ground cumin
½ teaspoon smoked paprika
¼ teaspoon freshly squeezed lime juice
1 large iceberg lettuce leaf
1 ounce Cheddar cheese, shredded
1 tablespoon sliced jalapeño
1½ tablespoons red taco sauce

1. Preheat an outdoor grill or stovetop grill pan over high heat.
2. In a medium bowl, mix the beef, cumin, paprika, and lime juice until well combined. Form a patty that is oblong rather than circular. Be careful not to overwork the meat or pack the patty too tightly.
3. Grill the patty to the desired doneness, 2 minutes per side for medium-rare.
4. Place the lettuce on a plate and place the burger on the stem end. Top with the cheese, jalapeño, and taco sauce. Fold the lettuce over the burger—no bun required. Serve.

Mushroom and Chia Seed Turkey Burger on Eggplant

Serves 2

3 tablespoons macadamia nut oil, divided
2 (½-inch-thick) eggplant slices
6 ounces cremini mushrooms, cut into ¼-inch dice
coarse sea salt and freshly ground black pepper
¼ cup ricotta cheese
6 ounces ground turkey breast
1 large egg, lightly beaten
1 teaspoon dried basil
¼ teaspoon chia seeds
2 lettuce leaves (optional)
2 red onion slices (optional)

1. Preheat the oven to 450°F.
2. Drizzle a baking sheet with 1 tablespoon of the oil and lay the eggplant slices on it. Drizzle another tablespoon of the oil over the eggplant slices. Roast for 2 to 3 minutes, flip the eggplant slices over, and roast for another 2 to 3 minutes—you want these crisp-tender and not mushy. Transfer the eggplant slices to two plates.
3. Heat the remaining 1 tablespoon oil in a skillet over medium-high heat. Add the mushrooms and sauté for 3 to 5 minutes.

4. Drain the liquid, transfer the mushrooms to a medium bowl, and season with salt and pepper. Add the ricotta cheese, ground turkey, egg, basil, and chia seeds. Form two patties. Be careful not to overwork the meat or pack the patties too tightly.
5. Preheat an outdoor grill or stovetop grill pan over medium-high heat. Grill the burgers for 5 to 7 minutes on each side.
6. Place a lettuce leaf and a slice of red onion, if desired, on each eggplant slice and top with a burger. Serve.

Tuna Melt on Portobello with Broccoli Sprouts

Serves 1

½ teaspoon macadamia nut oil, divided
1 medium portobello mushroom cap
1 (5-ounce) can albacore tuna
2 tablespoons sour cream
½ teaspoon Dijon mustard
2 tablespoons chopped walnuts
2 tablespoons diced red onion
½ teaspoon ground turmeric
½ teaspoon garlic powder
¼ teaspoon coarse sea salt, plus more for sprinkling
pinch freshly ground black pepper
pinch ground ginger
pinch ground coriander
¼ cup broccoli sprouts
1 slice Cheddar cheese

1. Preheat the broiler.
2. Drizzle ¼ teaspoon of the oil on a small baking sheet and place the mushroom, cap-side down, on it. Drizzle the mushroom cap with the remaining ¼ teaspoon oil and broil for 5 minutes. Turn the cap over and broil for another 5 minutes. Remove from the oven, return the mushroom to cap-side down, and leave on the baking sheet. Leave the broiler on.

3. Put the tuna in a bowl and use a fork to break up any large chunks. Add the sour cream, mustard, walnuts, onion, and seasonings and combine.

4. Top the mushroom cap with the tuna mixture. Lay the sprouts on top and then cover with cheese.

5. Broil until the cheese melts, about 1 minute.

6. Transfer the mushroom to a plate, sprinkle with salt, and serve.

Tri-Tip Gruyère Melt

Serves 2

3 tablespoons macadamia nut oil, divided
2 medium portobello mushroom caps
8 ounces tri-tip steak, thinly sliced
2 teaspoons Dijon mustard
2 handfuls kale, thinly sliced
1 avocado, peeled, pitted, and thinly sliced
2 ounces Gruyère cheese, sliced

1. Preheat the broiler.

2. Drizzle ½ tablespoon of the oil on a small baking sheet and place the mushrooms, cap-side down, on it. Drizzle the mushroom caps with another ½ tablespoon of the oil and broil for 5 minutes. Turn the caps over and broil for another 5 minutes. Remove from the oven, return the mushrooms to cap-side down, and leave on the baking sheet. Turn off the oven.

3. Meanwhile, heat the remaining 2 tablespoons oil in a medium skillet over high heat. Add the steak slices and cook for about 2 minutes on each side.

4. Spread the mustard evenly on the mushroom caps. Divide the steak, kale, and avocado evenly between the mushroom caps. Top with the cheese.

5. Place the baking sheet back in the cooling oven and allow the cheese to melt and the kale to wilt, about 2 minutes. Transfer the mushrooms to plates and serve.

Main Courses

Adobo Chicken with Mushrooms

Serves 4

4 bone-in, skin-on chicken breast halves
coarse sea salt and freshly ground black pepper
3 tablespoons salted grass-fed butter, divided
8 ounces oyster mushrooms, trimmed
8 ounces shallots, peeled and coarsely chopped
3 cups chicken broth
½ cup heavy cream
1 tablespoon coconut flour
½ teaspoon adobo paste
⅓ cup chopped fresh dill
3 bacon slices, cut into ½-inch pieces and cooked

1. Season the chicken with salt and pepper.
2. Melt 2 tablespoons of the butter in a large skillet over medium-high heat. Add the chicken, skin-side down, and cook, turning a few times, until browned all over, 10 to 12 minutes. Transfer the chicken to a plate.
3. Melt the remaining 1 tablespoon butter in the same skillet over medium heat. Add the mushrooms and shallots and season with salt. Cook, stirring and scraping up the browned bits, until golden brown in places, 8 to 10 minutes.
4. Add the broth and cream and bring to a boil. Return the chicken, skin-side up, and the accumulated juices to the skillet. Cover, decrease the heat, and simmer for 6 minutes. Stir.
5. Remove 3 tablespoons of the hot liquid from the skillet and transfer to a small cup. Whisk in the coconut flour. Pour this mixture and the adobo paste into the skillet and stir to mix well. Cover and cook for an additional 6 minutes.
6. Uncover and simmer until thickened, 2 to 3 minutes. Stir in the dill, top with the bacon, and serve.

Grilled Cashew Chicken

Serves 4

1 cup roasted, salted cashews
6 tablespoons chopped fresh cilantro with some stems, divided
4 garlic cloves, roughly chopped
2 jalapeños, seeded and sliced
¼ cup macadamia nut oil
2 tablespoons water
2 tablespoons tamari
juice of 1 lime
kosher salt and freshly ground black pepper
3 pounds bone-in, skin-on chicken thighs and/or drumsticks
lime wedges, for garnish (optional)

1. In a food processor, combine the cashews, 2 tablespoons of the cilantro, garlic, jalapeños, oil, water, tamari, and lime juice. Pulse until smooth, scraping down the sides as necessary. Taste and season with salt and pepper.

2. Season the chicken all over with salt and pepper. Smear on enough cashew mixture to thoroughly coat each piece. Reserve any remaining mixture. Let the chicken marinate at room temperature while you preheat an outdoor grill or broiler.

3. Grill the chicken or broil it on a baking sheet, turning frequently, until it is crisp and golden on the outside and cooked on the inside, 20 to 30 minutes.

4. Sprinkle the chicken with the remaining cilantro and serve with the remaining cashew mixture and lime wedges, if desired.

NOTE
Try serving this recipe with Frisée and Radicchio Salad with Mustard Vinaigrette (page 199).

Chinese-Style Chicken with Cashews

Serves 4

⅓ cup coarsely chopped cashews
2 tablespoons macadamia nut oil
1 pound boneless, skinless chicken breast, cut lengthwise into
    thin strips
2 cups julienned red bell pepper
1 teaspoon minced garlic
½ teaspoon minced fresh ginger
1 teaspoon tamari
1 head red leaf lettuce, chopped
3 tablespoons thinly sliced scallions

1. Heat a large skillet over medium-high heat. Add the cashews and cook until lightly toasted, stirring and tossing frequently—do not let them burn. Transfer to a bowl and set aside.
2. Add the oil to the same skillet, swirling to coat. Add the chicken and sauté until lightly browned, about 2 minutes. Transfer the chicken to a separate bowl and set aside.
3. Add the bell pepper to the skillet and sauté for 2 minutes, stirring occasionally. Add the garlic, ginger, and tamari and cook for 1 minute. Return the chicken to the skillet and cook for 1 minute more.
4. Divide the lettuce evenly among four plates. Top with the chicken and vegetables, sprinkle with the cashews and scallions, and serve.

Chicken and Avocado Salad with Lime Mayonnaise

Serves 4

FOR THE SALAD
1 (2¾-pound) chicken
1 teaspoon whole black peppercorns

8 garlic cloves, unpeeled
1 medium fennel bulb, with leaves
coarse sea salt
2 scallions, thinly sliced
1 avocado, peeled, pitted, and cut into ½-inch dice
1 tablespoon freshly squeezed lime juice

FOR THE LIME MAYONNAISE
1 large egg yolk
2 tablespoons freshly squeezed lime juice, or more to taste,
   divided
1 tablespoon Dijon mustard
1 small garlic clove, minced
coarse sea salt and freshly ground black pepper
¾ cup macadamia nut oil
½ avocado, peeled and pitted
¼ cup plus 2 tablespoons sour cream

1. To make the salad, put the chicken in a large stockpot and add the peppercorns and whole garlic cloves. Cut the fennel bulb into ¼-inch dice and reserve ½ cup; add the remainder to the pot. Chop the fennel leaves and reserve 2 tablespoons; add the remainder to the pot.

2. Add just enough water to cover the chicken and season generously with salt. Bring to a boil over medium-high heat, then decrease the heat to a simmer. Cook until the chicken juices run clear when sliced at a joint, 20 to 25 minutes.

3. Transfer the chicken to a plate and allow to cool completely. Reserve the broth for another use.

4. Remove the meat from the chicken, discarding the skin and bones. Cut the meat into ½-inch pieces. Transfer to a large bowl and add the scallions and the reserved diced fennel bulb and leaves.

5. Add the avocado. Sprinkle with the lime juice and toss gently to mix. Set aside.

6. To make the lime mayonnaise, in a small bowl whisk together the egg yolk, 1 tablespoon of the lime juice, mustard, garlic, and a large pinch each of salt and pepper. Beginning with a drop at a time,

whisk in the oil. As it emulsifies, add more oil in a slow, steady stream. (This step can also be done in a blender, but you have better control of the speed by hand.)

7. When all the oil is incorporated and the mixture is thick, press the avocado half through a sieve into the mixture. Add the remaining 1 tablespoon lime juice and the sour cream and whisk to blend. Season to taste with salt, pepper, and additional lime juice, if desired—it should be highly seasoned.

8. Fold ⅓ cup of the mayonnaise into the chicken salad. There should be just enough mayo to coat the chicken; add more to your desire. (Reserve the remaining mayonnaise in a covered container in the refrigerator for up to 3 days.) Cover and refrigerate for at least 1 hour before serving.

Stuffed Chicken with Squash Ribbons

Serves 6

FOR THE STUFFED CHICKEN
8 ounces mozzarella cheese, finely diced
½ cup pesto
6 boneless, skinless chicken breasts
1 cup finely grated Parmesan cheese
3 large eggs
¼ teaspoon cayenne pepper
coarse sea salt and freshly ground black pepper, to taste
3 tablespoons macadamia nut oil

FOR THE SQUASH RIBBONS
1 pound zucchini
1 pound yellow squash
¼ cup chicken broth
coarse sea salt and freshly ground black pepper
½ cup pesto
½ cup pine nuts, toasted
fresh basil leaves

1. To make the stuffed chicken, in a medium bowl mix the mozzarella and pesto.
2. Remove the tenders from the chicken breasts and reserve. Carefully insert the tip of a paring knife into the thickest part of the breast to form a pocket. Fill each pocket with an equal amount of the mozzarella mixture, then slide the reserved tender into the opening to seal it. Place the stuffed chicken on a plate, cover with plastic wrap, and chill for at least 4 hours and preferably overnight.
3. Preheat the oven to 350°F.
4. In a medium bowl, whisk together the Parmesan, eggs, cayenne, and salt and black pepper to form a thick mixture.
5. Heat the oil in a large skillet over medium-high heat.
6. Coat the stuffed breasts with the Parmesan mixture and place in the skillet. Immediately transfer the skillet to the oven. Bake until the chicken is cooked through, about 30 minutes.
7. Meanwhile, to make the squash ribbons, slice the zucchini and yellow squash into thin ribbons with a mandoline.
8. Bring the broth to a simmer in a large saucepan, add the ribbons, and season with salt and pepper. Sauté until cooked through, about 4 minutes. Add the pesto and pine nuts and toss to combine.
9. Divide the squash ribbons among six plates, add a stuffed chicken breast to each, and garnish with fresh basil leaves. Serve.

Chicken Ragout with Shirataki Noodles

Serves 4

2 tablespoons macadamia nut oil
1 small onion, finely chopped
1 celery stalk (including leaves), finely chopped
8 ounces shiitake mushrooms
2 medium carrots, peeled and finely chopped
coarse sea salt and freshly ground black pepper
1 pound ground chicken

12 ounces shirataki noodles
¾ cup heavy cream
freshly grated Parmesan cheese
4 fresh basil leaves

1. Heat the oil in a large skillet over medium-high heat. Add the onion, celery, mushrooms, and carrots and season with salt and pepper. Cook, stirring occasionally, until softened, 5 to 7 minutes.
2. Add the chicken and season with salt and pepper. Cook, breaking up the chicken into bite-size pieces, until no longer pink, 3 to 4 minutes.
3. Stir in the shirataki noodles and cook for 2 minutes. Add the cream and simmer until thickened, 12 to 15 minutes.
4. Divide the chicken and noodles among four plates, top with Parmesan and fresh basil, and serve.

Chicken Pesto

Serves 1

FOR THE PESTO
3 cups packed fresh cilantro
½ cup chopped fresh parsley
4 garlic cloves, peeled
¾ cup grated Parmesan cheese
½ cup extra virgin olive oil
¼ cup pine nuts

FOR THE CHICKEN
1 tablespoon balsamic vinegar
6 ounces boneless, skinless chicken breast, cut into strips
garlic powder
coarse sea salt
2 tablespoons macadamia nut oil, divided
1 cup chopped broccoli florets
1 teaspoon minced garlic
3 cups mixed baby greens

1. To make the pesto, combine all the ingredients in a food processor or blender. Blend to a smooth paste.
2. To make the chicken, mix 2 tablespoons of the pesto with the vinegar and set aside.
3. Season the chicken with garlic powder and salt.
4. Heat 1 tablespoon of the oil in a large wok over medium-high heat. Add the chicken in single strips and cook for about 1 minute on each side. Transfer the chicken to a plate.
5. Add the remaining 1 tablespoon oil to the wok. Add the broccoli and garlic and cook until the broccoli is bright green and crisp-tender, 2 to 3 minutes.
6. Return the chicken to the skillet. Add 2 tablespoons of the pesto-vinegar sauce and toss. Remove the wok from the heat.
7. Put the greens in a serving bowl. Add the remaining pesto-vinegar sauce to the greens and toss. Spoon the chicken and vegetables over the greens and serve.

NOTE

This recipe uses cilantro and parsley, so it isn't a classic pesto. If you don't like cilantro, simply use basil instead. This recipe makes enough pesto for multiple dishes, so use what you need for this recipe and store the leftovers in a covered container in the refrigerator for up to 3 days.

Chili, Garlic, and Basil Chicken over Shirataki Noodles

Serves 1

1½ teaspoons macadamia nut oil, divided
2½ teaspoons chili garlic sauce, divided
1½ teaspoons freshly squeezed lemon juice
6 ounces boneless, skinless chicken breast, cut into strips
2 ounces shirataki noodles
macadamia nut oil spray
1 clove garlic, peeled and crushed
½ cup diced red onion

4 asparagus spears, tops only (about 1 inch)
8 fresh basil leaves, slivered

1. Whisk together ½ teaspoon of the oil, 2 teaspoons of the chili garlic sauce, and the lemon juice in a small bowl. Set aside.
2. In a separate bowl, toss the chicken with the remaining ½ teaspoon chili garlic sauce. Set aside.
3. Pour the remaining 1 teaspoon oil into the bottom of a salad bowl and spread evenly; toss in the shirataki noodles.
4. Heat a large nonstick wok over medium-high heat. Spray the pan with a little macadamia nut oil. Add the garlic, onion, and asparagus. Cook until the onion is crisp-tender and the asparagus is bright green, about 5 minutes. Push the veggies to one side of the pan.
5. Respray the pan and add the chicken in a single layer. Cook for about 2 minutes on each side. Push the vegetables back into the center, add the sauce mixture, and thoroughly mix.
6. Spoon the chicken and vegetables over the noodles, top with the basil, and serve.

Chili-Glazed Chicken Drumsticks with Slaw

Serves 4

8 chicken drumsticks (about 2 pounds)
coarse sea salt and freshly ground white pepper
2 teaspoons sambal oelek or any chili paste
½ head napa cabbage, shredded
3 medium carrots, peeled and shredded
4 ounces shiitake mushrooms, stemmed and thinly sliced
3 tablespoons freshly squeezed lime juice
1 tablespoon toasted sesame oil
⅓ cup chopped fresh cilantro, plus more for garnish

1. Preheat the oven to 375°F. Line a rimmed baking sheet with parchment paper.

2. Place the chicken on the prepared baking sheet; season with salt and pepper.

3. Brush each drumstick with chili paste. Bake until just cooked through, about 45 minutes. Reserve the juices.

4. While the chicken is cooking, combine the cabbage, carrots, mushrooms, lime juice, oil, and cilantro in a large mixing bowl. Season with salt and pepper. Toss until thoroughly combined. Set aside.

5. Divide the slaw among four plates. Place two drumsticks on each bed of slaw and drizzle the reserved juices on top. Serve.

Roasted Mustardy Chicken

Serves 4

1 large onion, peeled and sliced
8 ounces white mushrooms, peeled and halved
12 ounces Brussels sprouts, trimmed and halved
8 thyme sprigs, divided
3 tablespoons macadamia nut oil, divided
½ teaspoon dried oregano
coarse sea salt and freshly ground black pepper
1 (3½-pound) chicken, at room temperature
2 lemons, halved
¼ cup Dijon mustard

1. Preheat the oven to 450°F.

2. In a 9 × 12-inch glass baking dish, toss together the onion, mushrooms, Brussels sprouts, 3 of the thyme sprigs, 2 tablespoons of the oil, and the oregano. Season with salt and pepper and spread into an even layer.

3. Season the chicken cavity with salt and pepper and stuff the lemon halves and remaining 5 thyme sprigs into the cavity.

4. Rub the remaining 1 tablespoon oil on the outside of the chicken, brush it with the mustard, and season with salt and pepper. Place the chicken on top of the vegetables and roast for 20 minutes.

5. Decrease the temperature to 375°F and roast until a meat thermometer inserted into the thickest part of a thigh registers 165°F, about 45 more minutes.
6. Transfer the chicken to a carving board and let rest for 15 minutes. Return the vegetables to the oven and continue roasting until tender and golden brown in places, about 10 to 15 minutes.
7. Carve the chicken and serve with the vegetables.

Spicy Roast Duck

Serves 4

1 (4-pound) duck
coarse sea salt and freshly ground black pepper
2 tablespoons harissa
1 tablespoon garlic powder
1 tablespoon onion powder
½ teaspoon cayenne pepper
½ teaspoon red pepper flakes

1. Preheat the oven to 425°F.
2. With a sharp knife, make tiny slits all over the duck breast and legs, going two-thirds of the way through the skin and fat but taking careful not to slice into the meat. Season the cavity and the outside of the duck with salt and pepper.
3. Mix the harissa and all the spices together in a small bowl. Rub the spice mixture all over the duck.
4. Place the duck on a rack in a roasting pan, breast-side up. Roast the duck for 15 minutes. Turn the duck breast-side down and roast for an additional 15 minutes. Decrease the temperature to 350°F. Turn the duck breast-side up again and roast for 20 minutes. Turn the duck one more time, breast-side down, and roast for a final 20 minutes.
5. Remove the roasting pan from the oven and allow the duck to rest for 10 minutes before carving and serving.

NOTE
This duck pairs well with Sautéed Collard Greens (page 254).

Turkey Fajitas

Serves 2

1 red bell pepper, seeded and thinly sliced
½ cup thinly sliced yellow onion
8 ounces turkey breast, cut into 1-inch slices
1½ teaspoons macadamia nut oil
1 teaspoon chili powder
1 teaspoon smoked paprika
½ teaspoon garlic powder
¼ teaspoon cayenne pepper
coarse sea salt, to taste
½ head green leaf lettuce, shredded
1 avocado, peeled, pitted, and sliced, for garnish
2 tablespoons sour cream, for garnish
2 tablespoons shredded Monterey Jack cheese, for garnish

1. Preheat the oven to 375°F.
2. In a medium bowl, combine the bell pepper, onion, turkey, oil, and spices and toss until the turkey and vegetables are well coated.
3. Spread out the mixture in a small baking pan. Cover the pan with aluminum foil and bake for 20 minutes.
4. Divide the lettuce between two plates. Top each plate with half of the turkey mixture, avocado, sour cream, and Monterey Jack. Serve.

Chinese Roast Pork

Serves 6

4 pounds boneless pork shoulder (butt)
2 cups water
2 scallions, trimmed and cut into 1-inch lengths
3 thin slices peeled fresh ginger
½ cup tamari
½ cup dry sherry
½ cup Chinese five-spice powder

1. Cut the meat (or have the butcher cut the meat) with the grain into 2 × 1-inch slices as long as the shoulder.

2. In a medium stockpot, combine the water, scallions, ginger, tamari, and sherry. Add the pork and stir to coat. Cover and simmer over medium-low heat for 15 minutes (do not stir). Turn off the heat and let the pork steep until the liquid is cool, about 1 hour.

3. Drain the pork in a colander, pat dry with paper towels, and set aside.

4. Arrange the oven racks in the top and bottom thirds of the oven and preheat the broiler. Line a roasting pan with foil and top with a roasting rack.

5. Rub the meat with the five-spice powder and place in a single layer on the rack in the roasting pan. Broil the pork on the top oven rack for 10 minutes, then turn the pork slices over, transfer the pan to the bottom oven rack, and continue broiling until the pork is slightly crispy and cooked through, 5 to 10 minutes more. Serve.

NOTE
I like to serve this with Stir-Fried Bok Choy with Ginger and Garlic (page 254).

Italian Roast Pork

Serves 10

1 (6- to 7-pound) boneless, skin-on pork shoulder
3 tablespoons kosher salt
4 garlic cloves, peeled and mashed to a paste
1 tablespoon chopped fresh rosemary
1 tablespoon freshly ground black pepper
1 tablespoon red pepper flakes
2 teaspoons fennel pollen or ground fennel seeds

1. Score the pork skin in a diamond pattern (or have the butcher do it), then flip the pork skin-side down. Massage the salt into the meat, then cover with the garlic, rosemary, black pepper, red pepper flakes, and fennel.

2.   Roll the pork tightly, with the skin facing out, and tie it securely with kitchen twine. Marinate, uncovered, in the refrigerator overnight so the skin dries out.
3.   Remove the pork from the refrigerator 2 hours before cooking.
4.   Preheat the oven to 200°F.
5.   Roast the pork until fork tender, 5 to 6 hours, then increase the temperature to 500°F and roast for 20 minutes more to crisp the skin.
6.   Set aside to rest for 45 minutes before slicing and serving.

NOTE
This is a dish my mother often made at Easter. Try serving it with Fried Marinated Zucchini (page 262).

Fresh Ham

Serves 12

1 (16-pound) fresh ham
1½ teaspoons kosher salt
1 tablespoon freshly ground black pepper
2 tablespoons fresh thyme
2 cups plus 2 tablespoons dry white wine, divided
½ cup water
¼ cup cream

1.   Preheat the oven to 425°F and place an oven rack in the lower third of the oven.
2.   Trim the skin and excess fat from the ham, leaving a layer of fat into which you will score a diamond pattern ½-inch deep and about 1½ inches wide.
3.   In a small bowl, rub the salt, pepper, and thyme and together with your fingers so the thyme becomes fragrant. Pat the mixture all over the ham and into the crevices.
4.   Place the ham, fat-side up, on a rack in a large roasting pan and roast for 30 minutes.
5.   Turn the heat down to 350°F. Pour 2 cups of the wine and the water into the pan and tent loosely with aluminum foil.

Continue roasting the ham, basting every half hour, until a meat thermometer inserted into the thickest part reads 155°F, about 3½ hours. Add more water to the pan if the pan juices start to scorch.

6. Transfer the ham to a carving board and allow to rest for 15 minutes before carving.

7. Meanwhile, pour the pan juices and the remaining 2 tablespoons wine into a small saucepan and simmer for 2 minutes. Turn off the flame, stir in the cream, and serve with the ham.

NOTE

Offer Zucchini-Basil Gratin (page 258) on the side.

Pork Stir-Fry with Broccolini and Peppers

Serves 1

1 (6-ounce) pork tenderloin, cut into strips
kosher salt
¼ teaspoon Chinese five-spice powder, or more to taste
3 tablespoons macadamia nut oil, divided
1½ cups shredded red cabbage
½ cup sliced yellow bell pepper
4 ounces broccolini, with stems, chopped
½ cup sliced red onion
1 teaspoon minced garlic

1. Season the pork with salt and the five-spice powder and set aside.

2. Heat 1 tablespoon of the oil in a wok over medium-high heat. Add the cabbage and a pinch of salt and stir-fry for 2 minutes. Transfer the cabbage to a serving plate.

3. Heat another tablespoon of oil in the wok. Add the bell pepper, broccolini, onion, and garlic. Cook until the pepper is lightly browned on the outside and almost tender, about 4 minutes. Transfer the vegetables to another plate.

4. Heat the remaining 1 tablespoon oil in the wok. Add the pork in one layer and cook for 2 minutes on each side. Return the

vegetables to the wok, stir together until heated through and mixed thoroughly, and pour over the cabbage. Serve.

Orange Beef and Broccoli

Serves 4

FOR THE BEEF
grated zest of 2 oranges
½ cup macadamia nut oil
1 (2-pound) flank steak
2 teaspoons kosher salt
2 teaspoons chili powder
1 teaspoon garlic powder
1 teaspoon onion powder
½ teaspoon dried oregano
½ teaspoon dried basil
½ teaspoon freshly ground black pepper

FOR THE BROCCOLI
2 heads broccoli, cut into large florets
½ cup macadamia nut oil, plus more for grilling
coarse sea salt and freshly ground black pepper
2 tablespoons finely chopped shallot
1 teaspoon Dijon mustard

1. To make the beef, combine ¾ of the orange zest, oil, and steak in a resealable plastic bag and mix well. Marinate in the refrigerator for at least 4 hours or preferably overnight.
2. When ready to cook, mix the rest of the seasonings in a small bowl.
3. Remove the steak from the marinade and rub with the seasoning mixture. Let the steak sit at room temperature for 1 hour. Strain the marinade through a fine-mesh sieve, reserving the zest. Set aside.
4. Heat an outdoor grill to high. Grill the steak to the desired doneness, about 5 minutes per side for medium-rare. Transfer the steak to a carving board and allow to rest for 10 minutes before slicing.

5. Meanwhile, to make the broccoli, bring a large pot of salted water to a boil over high heat and prepare an ice-water bath. Add the broccoli to the boiling water and cook for 1 minute. Drain and transfer the broccoli to the ice bath to cool.

6. Remove the broccoli from the ice bath and pat dry. Rub each floret with a little oil and season with salt and pepper.

7. Grill the broccoli until charred and tender, about 5 to 7 minutes.

8. Meanwhile, whisk together the shallot, mustard, ½ cup oil, remaining orange zest, and salt and pepper in a small bowl until emulsified.

9. Transfer the grilled broccoli to a large bowl and toss with the dressing.

10. Add the beef to the broccoli and mix thoroughly. Divide among four plates and serve.

Sriracha Steak on Swamp Cabbage

Serves 4

1 pound flank or skirt steak
¼ cup tamari
½ teaspoon toasted sesame oil
3 tablespoons rice wine vinegar, divided
1 English cucumber, thinly sliced
coarse sea salt
2 tablespoons macadamia nut oil
1 cup diced red onion
1 cup white button mushrooms, diced
1 cup dandelion greens
1 head swamp cabbage, leaves separated
sriracha, for drizzling

1. Combine the steak, tamari, sesame oil, and 1 tablespoon of the vinegar in a resealable plastic bag and marinate in the refrigerator for at least 4 hours or preferably overnight.

2. An hour before cooking, combine the sliced cucumber with a pinch of salt and the remaining 2 tablespoons vinegar in a small bowl and set aside.

3. Heat the macadamia nut oil in a cast-iron skillet over medium-high heat. Add the onion, mushrooms, and dandelion greens, season with salt, and cook until the greens are just wilted and the mushrooms are tender but not mushy, about 4 minutes.

4. Remove from the heat and pour into a colander set over a bowl to reserve the juices. Set the greens mixture aside. Place a few swamp cabbage leaves on each plate.

5. Return the skillet to medium-high heat. Cook the steak until a nice crust develops on the surface and the meat is firm but yielding to the touch, 3 to 4 minutes per side.

6. Transfer the steak to a carving board and slice thinly. Place a few slices on top of the swamp cabbage, top with some of the vegetable mixture, and finish with a drizzle of sriracha. Serve, with the reserved greens liquid as a dipping sauce.

Pepper Rib Eye Steak with Watercress and Purslane

Serves 4

2 (12-ounce) rib eye steaks, about 1 inch thick
1 tablespoon freshly ground black pepper
coarse sea salt
¼ cup dry red wine
2 tablespoons salted grass-fed butter
2 large bunches watercress, stemmed
2 large bunches purslane

1. Season the steaks on both sides with the pepper, lightly patting it in. Season with salt and set aside.

2. Heat a large cast-iron skillet over medium-high heat. When you can see heat rising from the skillet, sear the steaks in the dry skillet

without moving them until they are brown and crusty on the underside, about 4 minutes for medium-rare. Turn the steaks and sear for 4 minutes more, then transfer to a serving platter.

3. Pour off any excess fat, add the wine to skillet, and cook over low heat until the wine is reduced by half, stirring up any brown bits left behind by the steaks, about 1 minute. Pour the wine reduction over the steaks.

4. Wipe down the skillet and return to medium-low heat. Melt the butter in the skillet and add the watercress and purslane. Increase the heat to high and toss until the greens are wilted, 1 to 2 minutes. Season with salt.

5. Cut the steaks in half and arrange each half on a plate with a serving of the greens. Serve.

NOTE
Try serving this recipe with Braised Celery (page 258).

Steak Fajitas over Portobello Mushroom Strips

Serves 2

2 medium portobello mushroom caps
3 tablespoons macadamia nut oil, divided
12 ounces top round steak, cut into strips
⅛ teaspoon chili powder
⅛ teaspoon garlic powder
⅛ teaspoon onion powder
⅛ teaspoon red pepper flakes
⅛ teaspoon dried oregano
⅛ teaspoon smoked paprika
⅛ teaspoon ground cumin
coarse sea salt, to taste
1 cup sliced red onion
1 yellow bell pepper, seeded and sliced
1 poblano pepper, seeded and sliced
1 teaspoon minced garlic

4 tablespoons sour cream, for garnish
2 tablespoons finely chopped Fresno chiles, for garnish
fresh cilantro leaves, for garnish

1. Preheat the broiler.
2. In a bowl, toss the mushroom caps with 1 tablespoon of the oil to coat well. Place the mushrooms, cap-side up, on a baking sheet. Broil on each side for 5 minutes. Transfer to a plate.
3. In a medium bowl, toss the steak with the seasonings until well coated.
4. Heat the remaining 2 tablespoons oil in a wok or large skillet over medium-high heat. Add the onion, bell pepper, poblano, and garlic. Stir-fry until crisp-tender, about 3 minutes. Push the vegetables to one side of the wok and add the steak in a single layer. Cook until brown on the outside and pink in the center, about 1 minute on each side. Push the vegetables back to the center and combine.
5. Slice the mushroom caps and divide between two plates; top each with half of the steak and vegetable mixture. Garnish each serving with 2 tablespoons sour cream, 1 tablespoon chopped chiles, and cilantro and serve.

NOTE
All the seasonings, from the chili powder to the cumin, can be mixed together in equal quantities and stored in an airtight container for use in any Tex-Mex or Mexican-style dish.

Mother's Brisket

Serves 8

12 garlic cloves, minced
2 tablespoons finely chopped fresh rosemary
2 tablespoons freshly ground black pepper, or more to taste
1 tablespoon coarse sea salt, or more to taste
1 tablespoon red pepper flakes
1 tablespoon hot paprika
1 (8-pound) whole brisket, trimmed

¼ cup macadamia nut oil
2 large yellow onions, chopped
1 cup dry red wine

1. Preheat the oven to 450°F.
2. In a medium bowl, combine the garlic, rosemary, black pepper, salt, red pepper flakes, and paprika.
3. Place the brisket, fat-side up, in a large, deep roasting pan and rub it all over with the seasoning mixture. Roast the brisket for 20 minutes.
4. Meanwhile, heat the oil in a large skillet over medium-high heat. Add the onions and cook, stirring occasionally, until they soften, about 5 minutes. Strain and set aside.
5. Remove the brisket from the oven. Decrease the oven temperature to 325°F.
6. Pour the wine over the brisket, then add the onions. Cover the pan as tightly as you can with aluminum foil and roast for 3½ hours, turning the brisket once after 2 hours and again after another hour, each time ensuring that the foil is tightly on the pan.
7. Transfer the brisket to a cutting board. Let rest for 10 to 15 minutes. Carve the meat against the grain into thin slices.
8. Using a slotted spoon, transfer the onions and pan drippings to a blender, allowing the fat to fall through. Puree until smooth. Season to taste with salt and black pepper, then serve with the brisket.

NOTE
Brisket goes great with Green Bean Casserole (page 261).

Coconut Buffalo Curry

Serves 1

½ teaspoon macadamia nut oil
¼ cup diced white onion
½ teaspoon minced garlic
5 ounces ground bison

1 cup frozen vegetables (not peas, carrots, or corn—try broccoli, peppers, or anything else you like)

2 tablespoons tamari

1 tablespoon sriracha

1 tablespoon unsweetened shredded coconut flakes

1 teaspoon curry powder

½ teaspoon ground ginger

¼ teaspoon coarse sea salt

1 large egg

2 large egg whites

1. Heat the oil in a large sauté pan over medium heat. Add the onion and garlic and sauté until the onion starts to caramelize, 5 to 7 minutes.
2. Add the bison and break it up with a spoon as it cooks.
3. Once the meat starts to brown, stir in the frozen vegetables. Cover and cook for 3 minutes. Uncover and continue to cook, stirring for 2 more minutes.
4. Add the tamari, sriracha, coconut, curry powder, ginger, and salt.
5. Make a hole in the center of the bison mixture, revealing the bottom of the pan, and in it carefully crack the egg and add the egg whites. Scramble the eggs in the hole, then incorporate the scrambled eggs into the rest of the dish.
6. Transfer to a plate and serve.

Crispy Lamb with Cumin

Serves 4

1 small egg white

1 tablespoon dry sherry

1 tablespoon coconut flour

1 teaspoon coarse sea salt, or more to taste

½ teaspoon freshly ground black pepper

1 pound boneless lamb leg or shoulder, cut into ½ × 2-inch strips

3 tablespoons macadamia nut oil, divided

2 tablespoons cumin seeds, lightly cracked in a mortar

2 tablespoons dried red chiles
4 scallions, white and green parts only, cut on the diagonal into
1-inch lengths
toasted sesame oil, for drizzling

1. In a large bowl, whisk together the egg white, sherry, flour, salt, and pepper. Add the lamb strips and set aside to marinate for 1 hour.
2. Heat a large wok or skillet over high heat until a drop of water sizzles on contact. Swirl 1½ tablespoons of the macadamia nut oil into the wok and carefully add the lamb in a single layer. Let it sear for a moment, then stir-fry just until the lamb is no longer pink, 4 to 6 minutes. Transfer to a plate. (If your wok isn't big enough, this can be done in two batches, but you will need more oil.)
3. Swirl the remaining 1½ tablespoons oil into the empty wok, add the cumin seeds and chiles, and stir-fry for a few seconds, just until the cumin seeds start to pop. Press the chiles against the side of the wok to char their skins.
4. Add the scallions and stir-fry for 1 minute. Return the lamb to the wok and stir-fry until it is cooked through, about 2 minutes more.
5. Turn off the heat, sprinkle the stir-fry with salt and a few drops of sesame oil, and serve immediately.

Moroccan Leg of Lamb

Serves 8

1 (10-pound) bone-in leg of lamb, trimmed of fat and membrane
1 teaspoon kosher salt
1 teaspoon freshly ground black pepper
⅓ cup macadamia nut oil
⅓ cup freshly squeezed lemon juice
1 tablespoon grated lemon zest
2 tablespoons minced garlic
1 tablespoon harissa, plus more for serving
1 teaspoon whole coriander seeds, toasted and crushed
½ teaspoon ground cumin
Mint Dressing (page 265)

1. Score the meaty side of the lamb in a diamond pattern with ¼-inch-deep cuts about 1½ inches apart (or have the butcher do this). Season with salt and pepper and place it, scored-side up, in a large roasting pan.

2. In a small bowl, whisk together the oil, lemon juice and zest, garlic, harissa, coriander seeds, and cumin. When emulsified, pour the mixture over the lamb and massage it into the crevices. Cover the pan with aluminum foil and refrigerate for 2½ hours, or preferably overnight.

3. Remove the pan from the refrigerator 1½ hours before cooking; remove the foil and allow the lamb to come to room temperature; in the last 15 minutes, preheat the oven to 450°F.

4. Place the (uncovered) pan on the middle oven rack and immediately turn the heat down to 350°F. Roast, basting the lamb with the pan juices every half hour, until a meat thermometer inserted into the thickest part reads 130°F, about 1½ hours.

5. Remove from the oven, tent loosely with foil, and let rest for 15 minutes before carving.

6. Serve with extra harissa and mint dressing.

NOTE
Try serving this recipe with Sugar Snap Peas with Horseradish (page 257).

Roast Leg of Veal with Sausage Stuffing

Serves 8

FOR THE SAUSAGE STUFFING
4 Italian sweet sausages, removed from their casings
8 ounces ricotta cheese
½ onion, chopped
2 celery stalks, chopped
1 teaspoon coarse sea salt
½ teaspoon dried thyme
½ teaspoon dried sage

¼ cup heavy cream, as needed
½ cup grated Parmesan cheese, as needed

FOR THE VEAL

1 (5-pound) boned veal leg (have your butcher do this)
6 bacon slices
2 tablespoons macadamia nut oil
1 cheese and parsley sausage wheel, about 1 pound, taken apart
    and cut into 3-inch pieces
coarse sea salt and freshly ground black pepper

1. Preheat the oven to 325°F.
2. To make the stuffing, heat a medium saucepan over medium heat. Add a small amount of water and the sausage and cook, breaking up the meat with a spoon, until no longer pink, 5 to 6 minutes.
3. Drain the sausage and transfer it to a medium bowl. Mix it with the ricotta. Add the onion, celery, and seasonings, and just enough cream and Parmesan to bind the mixture.
4. Fill the meat cavity with the sausage mixture, then partially close the opening with 2 or 3 skewers laced with twine. Lay the bacon slices over the top of the meat.
5. Roast, uncovered, for 2 hours.
6. Meanwhile, heat the oil in a medium skillet over medium-high heat. Add the sausage wheel pieces and sear for about 3 minutes on each side. Add the sausage to the roasting pan, along with the skillet juices. Remove and reserve the bacon. Sprinkle the meat with salt and pepper. Roast for 1 more hour.
7. Meanwhile, cut the bacon into 1-inch pieces and sear in the same skillet until crispy. Scatter the bacon pieces in the roasting pan and continue roasting until a meat thermometer registers 170°F at the thickest part, about 30 minutes more (I actually remove mine at 160°F since the meat will continue to cook when removed from the oven).
8. Remove from the oven, tent loosely with foil, and let rest for 15 minutes before carving. Serve.

NOTE

For an impressive dinner, serve this dish with Whole Roasted Cauliflower with Green Herb Sauce (page 259).

Chia Seed Meatballs

Makes 4

8 ounces ground beef
1 large egg
½ cup grated Parmesan cheese
1 garlic clove, minced
1 teaspoon dried Italian herbs
1 teaspoon coarse sea salt
½ teaspoon freshly ground black pepper
1 tablespoon chia seeds
2 teaspoons avocado oil

1. Combine all the ingredients except the oil in a large bowl and mix well. Let rest for 10 minutes.
2. Heat the oil in a small skillet over medium heat. Shape the meat mixture into four balls. Add to the skillet and cook until brown on all sides, about 4 to 6 minutes. Serve.

Pizza with Chia Seed Meatballs and Red Pepper Sauce

Serves 2

FOR THE PIZZA CRUST
1 head cauliflower, cored
½ cup shredded mozzarella
¼ cup grated Parmesan cheese
½ teaspoon dried oregano
½ teaspoon kosher salt
¼ teaspoon garlic powder
2 large eggs, lightly beaten

FOR THE PIZZA
½ cup Red Pepper Sauce (page 266)
1 recipe Chia Seed Meatballs (page 235), thinly sliced

1. Preheat the oven to 400°F. Line a baking sheet with parchment paper.
2. To make the crust, break the cauliflower into florets and pulse in a food processor until about the size of couscous. In a medium pot, bring an inch of water to a boil over medium-high heat. Add a steamer basket, transfer the cauliflower to the steamer basket, and steam until tender, about 3 minutes. Drain well (I like to put it on a clean dishtowel to get all the moisture out). Let cool.
3. Transfer the cauliflower to a medium bowl and add the mozzarella, parmesan, oregano, salt, garlic powder, and eggs. Mix well. Transfer the mixture to the center of the prepared baking sheet and spread it into a circle, resembling a pizza crust. Turn the temperature down to 350°F. Bake for 20 minutes, then remove from the oven.
4. Spread the red pepper sauce all over the cauliflower crust, place the sliced meatballs evenly around the crust, and bake for 10 minutes more. Slice and serve.

NOTE
The cauliflower crust in this recipe can be used for any pizza—just use your imagination for the toppings, picking more alkaline foods and foods for your dieting type.

Pizza Siciliano with Sardines, Anchovy Paste, and Broccoli Sprouts

Serves 2

1 recipe cauliflower pizza crust (page 235)
1 tablespoon anchovy paste
1 (4-ounce) can sardines packed in olive oil
½ cup broccoli sprouts

1. Preheat the oven to 400°F. Line a baking sheet with parchment paper.
2. Spread the pizza crust mixture into a circle on the prepared baking sheet. Turn the temperature down to 350°F. Bake for 20 minutes, then remove from the oven.

3. Spread the anchovy paste all over the pizza crust, evenly place the sardines around the crust, and bake for 10 minutes more.
4. Top with the broccoli sprouts, slice, and serve.

Vegetable Lasagna

Serves 8

3 large zucchini, trimmed
1 teaspoon coarse sea salt
1 recipe Red Pepper Sauce (page 266)
1 (10-ounce) package frozen spinach, thawed and squeezed dry
1½ cups shredded carrots
2 large eggs
1 teaspoon dried oregano
1 tablespoon dried parsley
1½ cups ricotta cheese
fresh basil leaves
3 cups shredded mozzarella cheese, divided

1. Cut the zucchini in half crosswise, then lengthwise into ¼-inch-thick slices. Place the zucchini slices in a single layer on a large baking sheet. Sprinkle with salt and let rest for 10 minutes.
2. Heat a grill pan over medium-high heat and grill the zucchini slices on each side until tender, 1 to 2 minutes per side. Transfer to paper towels and set aside.
3. Preheat the oven to 350°F.
4. In a medium bowl, combine the red pepper sauce, spinach, and carrots. Mix well and set aside.
5. In a separate medium bowl, beat the eggs lightly. Add the oregano, parsley, and ricotta. Mix well.
6. To assemble, spread ¼ cup of the sauce mixture in a 9 × 13-inch baking dish. Top with one-third of the zucchini slices, in a single layer. Spread half of the ricotta mixture on top, then add half of the remaining sauce mixture. Scatter some fresh basil leaves on top and then sprinkle with 1 cup of the mozzarella.

7.   Repeat the layers with the remaining ingredients, topping the third
     and final layer of zucchini with the remaining 1 cup mozzarella
     and several fresh basil leaves.

8.   Cover with aluminum foil and bake for 20 minutes. Remove the
     foil and bake for another 15 minutes. Let cool on a wire rack for at
     least 10 minutes before cutting and serving.

Zucchini Pasta with Greens and Goat Cheese

Serves 4

4 zucchini
2 tablespoons macadamia nut oil, divided
2 garlic cloves, minced
1 tablespoon capers, drained
½ teaspoon red pepper flakes
¼ teaspoon freshly ground black pepper
½ cup chopped watercress
½ cup chopped fresh parsley
½ cup chopped fresh basil
¼ cup chopped walnuts, for garnish
⅓ cup grated Parmesan cheese, for garnish
⅓ cup goat cheese, for garnish

1.   Use a julienne peeler, mandoline, or spiralizer to cut the zucchini
     into "noodles."

2.   Heat 1 tablespoon of the oil in a large skillet over medium heat.
     Add the garlic and sauté until fragrant, about 1 minute.

3.   Add the zucchini noodles, capers, red pepper flakes, and black
     pepper. Cook until the zucchini is tender, about 2 minutes (do not
     overcook). Remove from the heat.

4.   Heat the remaining 1 tablespoon oil in a separate skillet over high
     heat. Add the watercress, parsley, and basil and wilt for about 1 minute.

5.   In a bowl, toss together the wilted greens and the zucchini mixture.
     Divide among four plates or shallow bowls.

6.   Garnish each serving with walnuts, Parmesan, and goat cheese and
     serve.

NOTE

As an option, you can add a soft-cooked egg to the top of each plate by simply cracking the eggs into the skillet you used for the greens (adding additional oil if necessary) and cooking until the whites are set and the outer edges start to curl up.

Turmeric Cauliflower Bowl

Serves 4

1 head cauliflower, cut into florets
3 tablespoons plus ¼ cup macadamia nut oil, divided
½ teaspoon curry powder
½ teaspoon ground turmeric
¼ teaspoon coarse sea salt
¼ teaspoon freshly ground black pepper
1 (½-inch) piece fresh ginger, peeled and minced
2 tablespoons freshly squeezed lemon juice
1 teaspoon Dijon mustard
¼ teaspoon red pepper flakes
½ cup pecans, toasted
½ cup chopped purslane

1. Preheat the oven to 400°F.
2. In a large mixing bowl, toss the cauliflower with 2 tablespoons of the oil, the curry powder, turmeric, salt, and pepper. Roast, tossing halfway, until the edges are golden brown, about 30 to 35 minutes.
3. Meanwhile, combine the ginger, lemon juice, mustard, and red pepper flakes in a small mixing bowl. Slowly whisk in the remaining ¼ cup macadamia nut oil to form an emulsion and set aside.
4. Remove the cauliflower from the oven and divide evenly among four bowls.
5. Drizzle the dressing over the bowls. Toss lightly, top with the toasted pecans and purslane and serve.

Fish and Seafood

Pistachio Smoked Salmon Rolls

Serves 4

1 pound smoked salmon, cut into ¼-inch-thick slices
1 cucumber, peeled and thinly sliced
1 12-ounce roll herbed goat cheese, cut into ⅛-inch slices
fresh thyme leaves
40 pistachios, crushed lightly

Top each salmon slice with a cucumber slice and a goat cheese slice. Sprinkle with thyme and pistachios. Roll them up and serve.

NOTE
This recipe makes a great hors d'oeuvres for a party.

Chinese-Style Sashimi

Serves 6

1 scallion, trimmed and minced
1 tablespoon tamari
1 teaspoon toasted sesame oil
coarse sea salt and freshly ground black pepper
1 pound skinless salmon, tuna, or wild striped bass fillet, very thinly sliced across the grain
cilantro sprigs, for garnish

1. Combine the scallion, tamari, sesame oil, and a pinch each of salt and pepper in a shallow bowl. Add the fish slices and toss gently to coat. Let stand for 10 minutes.
2. Transfer the fish to six chilled plates, garnish with cilantro, and serve.

Grilled Prawns
with Cauliflower Tabbouleh

Serves 6

FOR THE PRAWNS

**4 to 5 pounds fresh prawns (salt-water jumbo shrimp), shells and
  heads on**

½ cup macadamia nut oil

8 garlic cloves, minced

3 tablespoons za'atar spice blend

2 tablespoons red pepper flakes

coarse sea salt

FOR THE TABBOULEH

1 head cauliflower, cut into florets

3 tablespoons macadamia nut oil

1 large red onion, minced

3 garlic cloves, minced

coarse sea salt and freshly ground white pepper

grated zest and juice of 1 lemon

½ tablespoon za'atar spice blend

3 tablespoons chopped fresh parsley

3 tablespoons chopped fresh cilantro

2 tablespoons chopped fresh mint

fresh mint and cilantro leaves, for garnish

3 lemons, cut into 8 wedges each, for serving

1. In a large resealable bag or large bowl, toss the prawns with the
   oil, garlic, za'atar, and red pepper flakes. Cover and marinate in the
   refrigerator overnight.

2. To make the tabbouleh, pulse the cauliflower florets in a food
   processor until about the size of couscous.

3. Heat the oil in a large sauté pan over medium heat. Add the onion
   and garlic and sauté until translucent, about 5 minutes. Add the
   cauliflower, season with salt and white pepper, and sauté until just
   barely cooked, 3 to 4 minutes.

4. Transfer the cauliflower mixture to a large bowl and toss with the lemon zest and juice, za'atar, and chopped fresh herbs. Season to taste with salt and white pepper and set aside.

5. To cook the prawns, remove from the marinade and season liberally with salt. Preheat an outdoor grill or stovetop grill pan over high heat. Grill the prawns until cooked through, about 2 minutes per side.

6. Transfer to a serving plate and spoon the tabbouleh around the prawns. Garnish with the mint and cilantro leaves and serve with the lemon wedges.

Salmon-Stuffed Cabbage

Serves 4

1 medium head savoy cabbage
1 pound canned salmon
3 garlic cloves, peeled
½ cup chopped fresh parsley
½ cup watercress leaves
1½ tablespoons extra virgin olive oil
¼ teaspoon cayenne pepper
coarse sea salt
1½ tablespoons macadamia nut oil
1 large onion, peeled and chopped
freshly ground black pepper
¼ cup chicken broth
alfalfa sprouts, for garnish

1. Bring a large pot of salted water to a boil over high heat.

2. Meanwhile, remove enough outer leave of the cabbage to get 8 large, nearly perfect leaves. Use a paring knife to remove their thickest vein. Blanch the leaves in the boiling water until softened, about 1 minute. Remove and drain on paper towels.

3. Combine the salmon, garlic, parsley, watercress, olive oil, cayenne, and a large pinch of salt in a food processor. Pulse until minced and well combined but not pureed.

4. Spoon a portion of the salmon mixture on the lower third of each cabbage leaf, fold in the sides, and roll up. Be careful not to overstuff or roll too tightly.

5. Heat the macadamia nut oil in a large skillet over medium-high heat. Add the onion and sauté until it softens, about 5 minutes. Season with salt and pepper. Add the chicken broth and cook for another 5 minutes.

6. Carefully add the cabbage rolls, seam-side down, in a single layer and cover the skillet. Adjust the heat to a simmer and cook, turning once, until the rolls are firm, 10 to 15 minutes. (You may need to add a bit more broth.)

7. Place two cabbage rolls on each plate, drizzle with some pan juices, garnish with alfalfa sprouts, and serve.

NOTE
You can use cooked shrimp or ground beef in place of the salmon.

Monkfish Curry

Serves 4

FOR THE CURRY
4 tomatoes, roughly chopped
macadamia nut oil
½ teaspoon mustard seeds
½ teaspoon fenugreek seeds
2 curry leaves
1 (1-inch) piece ginger, peeled and julienned
1 onion, thinly sliced
½ teaspoon ground turmeric
1 cup hot water
4 teaspoons ground coriander
1 teaspoon chili powder
1 teaspoon ground cumin

FOR THE MONKFISH

1 tablespoon toasted sesame oil
1 tablespoon water
1 cup broccoli florets
½ large red bell pepper, cut into strips
½ cup Chinese long beans
1 garlic clove, minced
1 teaspoon minced fresh ginger
6 fresh shiitake mushrooms, cut into slivers
1 cup shredded Napa cabbage
⅓ cup cashews
3 tablespoons chicken broth
3 tablespoons tamari
1 (1-pound) monkfish fillet, cut into ½-inch pieces
¼ cup coconut milk
coarse sea salt
1 cup fresh cilantro leaves, chopped

1. To make the curry, in a blender, pulse the tomatoes into a puree and set aside.
2. In a cast-iron skillet over medium heat, heat enough oil to coat the bottom of the pan, then add the mustard seeds. Once the seeds are crackling, add the fenugreek seeds, followed by the curry leaves, julienned ginger, and sliced onion. Cook until the onion is golden, stirring occasionally.
3. Stir in the turmeric, then add the pureed tomatoes and hot water. Add the coriander, chili powder, and cumin. Partially cover the pan, turn up the heat, and let boil gently for 20 minutes.
4. Meanwhile, to make the monkfish, heat the sesame oil in a large skillet or wok over medium heat. Add the water, broccoli, bell pepper, beans, garlic, and ginger and stir-fry for 1 minute. Add the mushrooms, cabbage, and cashews and stir-fry for 2 minutes.
5. Whisk together the broth and tamari, add this to vegetables, and stir-fry for 2 minutes more.

6. Turn down the heat, add the monkfish, and simmer for 2 minutes, stirring gently. Add the coconut milk, season with salt, and bring the mixture back to a boil. Stir gently until everything is combined and the fish is cooked, then remove from the heat. Divide the spice mixture from steps 2 and 3 evenly among four bowls and top with the monkfish curry. Sprinkle with chopped cilantro, season with salt, and serve immediately.

Halibut with Salsa Fresca

Serves 4

2 ripe plum tomatoes, cored and chopped
½ large white onion, minced
½ cup roughly chopped fresh cilantro or parsley
juice of 3 or 4 limes
¼ habanero chile, seeded and minced
¼ jalapeño, seeded and minced
coarse sea salt
1½ pounds halibut
1 tablespoon avocado oil
freshly ground black pepper

1. Preheat the oven to 500°F.
2. In a medium bowl, toss together the tomatoes, onion, cilantro, lime juice, chiles, and jalapeño. Season with salt and set aside.
3. Rub the fish with the oil and season with salt and pepper. Place on a baking sheet and roast until cooked through, about 10 minutes.
4. Allow the fish to rest for 2 minutes, then plate and serve with the salsa.

NOTE
Try serving this recipe with Mustardy Asparagus (page 255).

Broiled Bluefish with Herbs

Serves 4

1 tablespoon minced garlic
3 tablespoons minced fresh rosemary
3 tablespoons minced fresh thyme
3 tablespoons freshly squeezed lemon juice, divided
1 teaspoon grated lemon zest
1 large egg yolk
1 teaspoon Dijon mustard
coarse kosher salt
¾ cup macadamia nut oil
2 Meyer lemons, cut into thin rounds
5 rosemary sprigs
5 thyme sprigs
4 (8-ounce) bluefish fillets
freshly ground white pepper

1. Using a mortar and pestle, pound the garlic, minced herbs, and 1 tablespoon of the lemon juice into a rough paste. Transfer to a bowl and add the remaining 2 tablespoons lemon juice, zest, egg yolk, mustard, and a pinch of salt.
2. Slowly whisk in the oil, increasing the speed to a slow, steady stream once the mayonnaise begins to emulsify. Whisk to the desired consistency and adjust the seasonings.
3. Preheat the broiler with the rack 6 inches from the heat.
4. Line a medium baking dish with the lemon slices and top with the herb sprigs. Lay the fish fillets, skin-side down, on top.
5. Slather the fillets with a thin layer of mayonnaise and broil for 8 to 12 minutes, depending on the thickness of the fish. Blues are done when the thickest part of the fillet flakes easily with a fork. Season with salt and white pepper and serve.

NOTE
I like to serve this bluefish with Roasted Broccolini (page 255).

Alaska King Crab Legs

Serves 8

8 tablespoons (1 stick) salted grass-fed butter
2 teaspoons white miso
2 tablespoons freshly squeezed Meyer lemon juice
4 pounds steamed Alaska king crab legs, thawed

1. Bring the butter to a simmer in a small saucepan over medium-low heat, occasionally skimming off the foam on the surface and letting the milk solids fall to the bottom.
2. Carefully pour the clarified butter into a small bowl, leaving behind the solids. Stir in the miso and lemon juice.
3. Serve the crab legs with the warm butter mixture.

NOTE
King crab legs are sold steamed and flash frozen. Thaw them in the refrigerator for at least 8 hours and up to one day before serving. I like to serve them with Creamed Brussels Sprouts with Pancetta (page 256).

Crusted Pike with Asparagus

Serves 2

2 tablespoons avocado oil
1 bunch asparagus, peeled and woody bottoms snapped off
coarse sea salt and freshly ground black pepper
½ cup almond meal
¼ teaspoon cayenne pepper
¼ teaspoon smoked paprika
2 walleyed pike fillets
2 tablespoons macadamia nut oil
2 quail eggs
1½ teaspoons grated Parmesan cheese
½ teaspoon freshly squeezed lemon juice

1. Preheat the broiler.

2. Heat the avocado oil in a large skillet over medium-high heat. Add the asparagus and season with salt and pepper. Sauté until crisp-tender, 10 to 12 minutes.

3. Meanwhile, in a shallow dish, combine the almond meal, cayenne, paprika, and salt and pepper to your liking. Coat the fish with the almond meal mixture.

4. Heat the macadamia nut oil in another large skillet over medium heat. Add the fish and cook until golden brown and cooked through, 3 to 4 minutes per side. Remove from the heat.

5. When the asparagus is done, remove the skillet from the heat, carefully crack the eggs over the asparagus, and broil for 1½ minutes. Remove and top with the grated Parmesan.

6. Drizzle the fish with the lemon juice, plate with the asparagus and eggs, and serve.

Razor Clams with Kielbasa

Serves 4

4 tablespoons macadamia nut oil, divided
1 large yellow onion, sliced
coarse sea salt and freshly ground black pepper
24 razor clams, cleaned
12 Manila clams, scrubbed
4 ounces kielbasa sausage, sliced
½ cup dry white wine
¼ cup tamari
1 tablespoon sherry vinegar
2 tablespoons minced scallion
1 tablespoon minced fresh ginger
2 jalapeños, finely chopped, for garnish

1. Heat 2 tablespoons of the oil in a large skillet over medium-high heat. Add the onion, season with salt and pepper, and sauté just until the onion softens, about 1 minute.

2. Add the clams and raise the heat to high; cook for 1 minute. Add the sausage and sauté for 1 minute more.

3. Add the wine, cover, and cook until the clams are tender, about 5 minutes. Discard any clams that do not open.

4. Meanwhile, in a small bowl, combine the remaining 2 tablespoons oil, tamari, vinegar, scallion, and ginger.

5. Divide the clams and sausage and their juices among four large soup bowls. Spoon some of the scallion-ginger sauce over each, garnish with jalapeños, and serve.

Grilled Swordfish

Serves 4

½ teaspoon chili powder
½ teaspoon ground ginger
1 teaspoon ground coriander
juice of 3 limes
1 cup macadamia nut oil
4 (8-ounce) swordfish steaks
coarse sea salt

1. In a small, dry sauté pan, toast the spices over medium heat. Stir in the lime juice and set aside to cool for 5 minutes. Whisk in the oil.

2. Place the swordfish steaks in a shallow dish and coat with the mixture. Cover and marinate in the refrigerator for 2 hours.

3. When ready to serve, preheat an outdoor grill to high. Sprinkle each side of the swordfish with salt and grill until just cooked through, 3 to 5 minutes per side depending on the thickness of the steak. Serve.

NOTE
Offer Garlicky Stir-Fried Chinese Long Beans (page 257) alongside.

Baked Salmon with Braised Fennel

Serves 4

4 (8-ounce) boneless, skinless salmon fillets
1 teaspoon ground sumac
coarse sea salt
extra virgin olive oil, for drizzling
3 fennel bulbs, 2 trimmed and cut into small wedges, 1 trimmed
**   and thinly sliced on a mandoline**
1 cup unsalted chicken broth
3 tablespoons macadamia nut oil, divided
2 shallots, sliced
1 cup dry red wine
3 tablespoons unsalted grass-fed butter, melted
4 ounces arugula
juice of ½ lemon
1½ teaspoons balsamic vinegar
freshly ground white pepper

1. Preheat the oven to 350°F. Line a baking sheet with aluminum foil.
2. Season both sides of the salmon fillets with the sumac and salt. Drizzle with olive oil and place on the prepared baking sheet. Bake the fillets for 8 minutes, turning once halfway through.
3. Meanwhile, combine the fennel wedges, chicken broth, and 1 tablespoon of the macadamia nut oil in a medium saucepan and season with salt. Cover and cook over medium heat until the fennel is tender, about 15 minutes. Remove the fennel from the liquid and set aside, covered to keep warm.
4. Combine the shallots and wine in a small saucepan over high heat. Cook until the liquid is reduced by a third, then strain through a fine-mesh sieve. Discard the solids and return the liquid to the pan. Decrease the heat and whisk in the butter.

5. In a medium bowl toss together the arugula and thinly sliced
   fennel. Drizzle with the lemon juice, balsamic vinegar, and
   remaining 2 tablespoons macadamia nut oil. Season with salt and
   white pepper.

6. Plate the salmon fillets and garnish each with some braised fennel
   wedges. Drizzle the sauce around the plate, add the arugula and
   sliced fennel atop the salmon, and serve.

Side Dishes

Stir-Fried Bok Choy with Ginger and Garlic

Serves 6

1 tablespoon macadamia nut oil
2 garlic cloves, minced
1 tablespoon minced fresh ginger
8 cups chopped bok choy
2 tablespoons tamari
coarse sea salt and freshly ground black pepper
1 teaspoon sesame seeds, toasted

1. Heat the oil in a large skillet over medium heat. Add the garlic and ginger and cook for 1 minute.
2. Add the bok choy and tamari and cook until the greens are wilted and the stalks are crisp-tender, 3 to 5 minutes. Season with salt and black pepper, sprinkle with the sesame seeds, and serve.

Sautéed Collard Greens

Serves 4

2½ pounds collard greens
1 tablespoon unsalted grass-fed butter
1 tablespoon macadamia nut oil
2 garlic cloves, minced
¼ teaspoon red pepper flakes
coarse sea salt and freshly ground black pepper
1 teaspoon freshly squeezed lemon juice, or to taste

1. Remove and discard the stems and center ribs of the collard greens. Cut the leaves into 1-inch pieces.
2. Bring a large pot of salted water to a boil over high heat. Cook the collards for 15 minutes, then drain in a colander, pressing out the excess liquid with the back of a wooden spoon.
3. In a 12-inch heavy-bottomed skillet, heat the butter and oil over medium-high heat until the foam subsides. Add the garlic,

collards, red pepper flakes, and salt and pepper to taste. Sauté the collard mixture until heated through, about 5 minutes.

4. Drizzle the collards with lemon juice and toss well. Serve.

Mustardy Asparagus

Serves 4

2 pounds jumbo asparagus, trimmed and bottoms peeled
2 tablespoons champagne vinegar
1 tablespoon Dijon mustard
½ teaspoon hot Chinese mustard
coarse sea salt and freshly ground black pepper
½ cup extra virgin olive oil

1. Bring a large pot of salted water to a boil over high heat. Prepare an ice-water bath.
2. Add the asparagus to the boiling water and blanch until tender, 3 to 4 minutes. Drain and transfer to the ice bath; when cool, drain on a paper towel–lined plate.
3. Whisk together the vinegar and mustards and season with salt and pepper. Whisking continuously, add the oil in a slow, steady stream until it emulsifies.
4. Transfer the asparagus to a platter and serve with the vinaigrette.

Roasted Broccolini

Serves 2

3 heads broccolini, cut into florets
2 tablespoons macadamia nut oil, divided
coarse sea salt and freshly ground black pepper
1 head garlic
1 teaspoon red pepper flakes
½ lemon
3 tablespoons grated Asiago cheese

1. Preheat the oven to 475°F.
2. In a medium bowl, toss the broccolini with 1 tablespoon of the oil and season with salt and pepper. Spread the broccolini on a baking sheet.
3. Halve the garlic head and drizzle with the remaining 1 tablespoon oil. Place the garlic halves on the baking sheet, face-side up. Sprinkle the red pepper flakes over the garlic and broccolini.
4. Roast until the broccolini is just slightly crispy, 20 to 25 minutes.
5. Squeeze the garlic clove out of the papery skin and distribute over the broccolini, or you can discard the garlic for a more subtle flavor.
6. Squeeze the lemon juice over the broccolini, sprinkle with grated Asiago, and serve.

Creamed Brussels Sprouts with Pancetta

Serves 4

2 tablespoons macadamia nut oil
3 ounces paper-thin pancetta slices, coarsely chopped
2 garlic cloves, minced
1 pound Brussels sprouts, trimmed and halved
freshly ground black pepper
½ cup heavy cream
½ cup grated Parmesan cheese
coarse sea salt

1. Heat the oil in a large heavy-bottomed or cast-iron skillet over medium heat. Add the pancetta and sauté until beginning to crisp, about 3 minutes. Add the garlic and sauté until pale golden, about 2 minutes. Remove the pancetta and garlic with a slotted spoon and transfer to a paper towel–lined plate.
2. Add the Brussels sprouts to the same skillet and sauté until heated through and beginning to brown, about 10 minutes. Season with pepper to taste.

3. Return the pancetta and garlic to the skillet and heat through for about 1 minute. Add the cream and bring to a boil, then decrease the heat to a brisk simmer.

4. Gently add the Parmesan and stir continuously until the mixture is thickened, about 5 minutes. Add salt, if necessary, and serve.

Garlicky Stir-Fried Chinese Long Beans

Serves 4

2 tablespoons macadamia nut oil
1 Szechuan red pepper, minced
1 tablespoon minced garlic
8 ounces Chinese long beans, cut into 2-inch pieces
1 tablespoon water
½ teaspoon coarse sea salt
1 teaspoon tamari

Heat the oil in a wok over medium-high heat. Add the Szechuan pepper and garlic and cook until the garlic begins to slightly brown, 1 to 2 minutes. Add the beans and water, cover, and steam until the beans are cooked through, about 5 minutes. Add the salt and tamari and serve.

Sugar Snap Peas with Horseradish

Serves 8

3 cups vegetable broth
¼ cup tamari
2 pounds sugar snap peas, trimmed
6 tablespoons (¾ stick) salted grass-fed butter
coarse sea salt and freshly ground black pepper
¼ cup grated fresh horseradish

1. Combine the broth and tamari in a deep skillet and cook over high heat until reduced to 1 cup, about 10 minutes.
2. Add the peas and stir frequently until they are bright green and tender and the liquid is reduced to a glaze, about 5 minutes.
3. Decrease the heat to medium and stir in the butter. Season with salt and pepper.
4. Transfer the peas to a warmed bowl and top with the horseradish. Serve.

Zucchini-Basil Gratin

Serves 6

1 tablespoon macadamia nut oil
2 pounds zucchini or yellow squash, thinly sliced crosswise
1 generous cup chopped fresh basil
¾ cup grated Gruyère cheese
1 cup heavy cream

1. Preheat the oven to 350°F. Place a rack in the lower third of the oven.
2. Oil a 9 × 13-inch baking dish and cover the bottom with a layer of zucchini slices. Sprinkle with some basil and Gruyère.
3. Repeat the layers until all the ingredients are used. Pour the heavy cream over the top.
4. Bake for 1 hour. Serve.

Braised Celery

Serves 4

1 large head celery
coarse sea salt and freshly ground white pepper
4 thyme sprigs
⅛ teaspoon cayenne pepper
3 tablespoons unsalted grass-fed butter
1 cup chicken broth
¼ cup macadamia nut oil

1. Preheat the oven to 375°F. Place a rack in the upper third of the oven.
2. Cut each celery stalk in half lengthwise and peel the large outer stalks with a vegetable peeler. Trim ¼ inch from the base and trim the tops so each stalk is about 12 inches long.
3. Arrange the celery in a single layer, peel-side up, in a 9 × 13-inch baking dish. Season liberally with salt and pepper, then add the thyme sprigs. Sprinkle on the cayenne and dot with butter. Pour in the broth and oil.
4. Cover the pan with aluminum foil and bake until the celery is knife tender, about 45 minutes. Turn the oven to broil.
5. Remove the foil and broil the celery until charred in spots, 5 to 10 minutes. Serve.

Whole Roasted Cauliflower with Green Herb Sauce

Serves 4

1 large head cauliflower, cored
¾ cup macadamia nut oil, divided
coarse sea salt and freshly ground black pepper
½ cup packed chopped fresh cilantro leaves and stems
½ cup packed chopped fresh parsley leaves
½ teaspoon minced garlic
1½ teaspoons Dijon mustard
2 tablespoons champagne vinegar

1. Preheat the oven to 450°F.
2. Brush the cauliflower all over with ¼ cup of the oil. Season with salt and pepper, then place it on a baking sheet. Put the baking sheet in the oven and immediately decrease the temperature to 400°F. Roast until golden brown and tender, about 1 hour.
3. Meanwhile, stir together the cilantro, parsley, garlic, mustard, vinegar, and remaining ½ cup oil in a small bowl to combine. Season with salt and pepper. Pour on top of the warm cauliflower and serve.

Roasted Cauliflower with Freekeh Pilaf

Serves 4

1 large head cauliflower, cut into florets
1 tablespoon macadamia nut oil, plus more for cauliflower
coarse sea salt and freshly ground black pepper
¼ cup slivered almonds
1¼ cups cracked freekeh
2 garlic cloves, minced
1/2 teaspoon coarse sea salt
1/4 teaspoon ground cumin
1/4 teaspoon ground coriander
3 cups vegetable broth
1 recipe Garlicky Tahini Sauce (page 269)
chopped fresh parsley, for garnish
crumbled feta cheese, for garnish
sesame seeds, for garnish

1. Preheat the oven to 425°F.
2. Toss the cauliflower florets with enough oil to cover them in a light, even layer. Season with salt and pepper and arrange the florets in a single layer on a large rimmed baking sheet. Roast, tossing halfway, until the florets are deeply golden on the edges, 30 to 35 minutes.
3. Meanwhile, warm 1 tablespoon oil in a cast-iron skillet over medium heat. Add the almonds and cook, stirring occasionally, until they're fragrant and turning golden on the edges, about 3 minutes.
4. Add the freekeh and sauté for 2 minutes, then add the garlic, salt, cumin, and coriander and sauté for 1 minute more.
5. Add the vegetable broth, increase the heat, and bring the mixture to a boil. Decrease the heat to medium-low, cover, and cook, stirring occasionally and decreasing the heat as necessary to maintain a gentle simmer, until the freekeh is tender to the bite, 20 to 25 minutes.
6. Drain off any excess liquid, cover, and set aside for 5 minutes. Fluff with a fork and season with salt and pepper.

7. Divide the freekeh among six plates and top with the roasted cauliflower. Drizzle the tahini sauce generously over each dish and then top with a sprinkling of parsley, feta, and sesame seeds. Serve.

Green Bean Casserole

Serves 8

1½ pounds green beans, trimmed and halved crosswise
2 tablespoons salted grass-fed butter, divided
3 onions, 2 thinly sliced and 1 coarsely chopped
1 teaspoon coarse sea salt, or more to taste
2 garlic cloves, minced
8 ounces button mushrooms, coarsely chopped
1 cup chicken broth
1 cup heavy cream
1 tablespoon coconut flour

1. Preheat the oven to 400°F.
2. Bring a large pot of salted water to a boil over high heat. Prepare an ice-water bath.
3. Add the beans to the boiling water and cook for 2 minutes. Drain and transfer to the ice bath.
4. Melt 1 tablespoon of the butter in a medium skillet over medium heat. Add the sliced onions, salt lightly, and cook until the onions are browned and caramelized, about 10 minutes.
5. Meanwhile, melt the remaining 1 tablespoon butter in a large skillet over medium heat. Add the chopped onion, garlic, mushrooms, and 1 teaspoon salt and cook for 10 minutes.
6. In a saucepan, bring the broth and cream to a simmer over medium heat. Add the flour and stir constantly for 2 minutes. Add the broth mixture to the mushroom mixture and bring to a boil, stirring until thickened.
7. Put the beans in a baking dish, add the mushroom mixture, and top with the caramelized onions. Bake until the onions crisp on the top and the bean mixture is bubbling, about 15 minutes. Serve.

Fried Marinated Zucchini

Serves 6

macadamia nut oil, for frying
6 zucchini, cut into ¼-inch-thick rounds
1 teaspoon coarse sea salt
2 garlic cloves, thinly sliced
¼ cup finely chopped fresh mint
¼ cup fresh watercress
⅔ cup white wine vinegar
extra virgin olive oil, for drizzling

1. Line a wire rack with paper towels.
2. In a medium cast-iron skillet, heat 2 inches of macadamia nut oil over medium heat. Fry the zucchini in small batches until golden brown and transfer to the rack to drain. Season with salt.
3. While the last batch of zucchini is cooling, combine the garlic, mint, watercress, and vinegar in a medium bowl.
4. Add the zucchini slices to the vinegar marinade and toss to coat. Cover and marinate overnight in the refrigerator.
5. When ready to serve, drizzle with olive oil.

Amaranth Tabbouleh

Serves 4

1½ cups cold water
½ cup whole-grain amaranth
½ cup drained canned chickpeas (garbanzo beans)
2 cups diced English cucumber
½ cup thinly sliced celery
½ cup finely chopped red onion
¼ cup chopped fresh mint
¼ cup chopped fresh parsley
¼ cup pine nuts, toasted

2 tablespoons macadamia nut oil
1 teaspoon grated lemon zest
2 tablespoons freshly squeezed lemon juice
¼ teaspoon kosher salt
¼ teaspoon red pepper flakes
1 cup (4 ounces) crumbled feta cheese
lemon wedges, for garnish

1. Combine the cold water and amaranth in a medium saucepan and bring to a boil over medium-high heat. Decrease the heat, cover, and simmer until the water is almost absorbed, about 20 minutes (it will have the appearance of mush).
2. While the amaranth cooks, combine the remaining ingredients except the feta and lemon wedges in a large bowl. Toss well.
3. Put the amaranth in a sieve and rinse under cold running water until room temperature; drain well, pressing with the back of a spoon. Add the amaranth to the vegetable mixture and toss to combine.
4. Add the feta and toss gently. Plate and garnish with lemon wedges to serve.

Cloud Bread

Serves 2

2 large eggs, separated
¼ cup heavy cream
⅛ teaspoon cream of tartar

1. Preheat the oven to 300°F.
2. In a small bowl, whisk together the egg yolks and cream. Transfer to a small baking dish.
3. In a separate bowl, beat the egg whites with the cream of tartar until they peak.
4. Carefully fold the egg whites into the egg yolk mixture.
5. Bake until the cloud bread is golden brown, about 30 minutes. Serve warm.

Condiments and Sauces

Mint Dressing

Makes 1 cup

2 cups tightly packed fresh mint leaves
2 tablespoons chopped shallot
1 small garlic clove, peeled
½ cup extra virgin olive oil
2 teaspoons red wine vinegar
½ teaspoon kosher salt, or more to taste
freshly ground black pepper

In a food processor, combine the mint, shallot, garlic, oil, vinegar, and salt and process until smooth. Season with more salt and pepper to taste.

NOTE
Mint and lamb make a classic pairing.

Aioli

Makes 1 cup

2 large garlic cloves, peeled
2 large egg yolks
¼ cup Fish Broth (page 186)
1½ teaspoons Dijon mustard
¾ teaspoon coarse sea salt
⅛ teaspoon cayenne pepper
½ cup macadamia nut oil
¼ cup extra virgin olive oil

Combine the garlic, egg yolks, broth, mustard, salt, and cayenne in a blender and puree until combined. While the machine is running, add the oils in a slow, steady stream until thick and emulsified.

Red Pepper Sauce

Makes 3 cups

12 red bell peppers
2 tablespoons macadamia nut oil, divided
¼ cup chopped onion
6 garlic cloves, minced
½ teaspoon anchovy paste (optional)
1 cup beef broth
1 cup chopped fresh basil
coarse sea salt and freshly ground black pepper

1. Preheat the oven to 500°F.
2. Place the bell peppers on a baking sheet and roast, turning them twice, until the skins are completely wrinkled and charred, 30 to 40 minutes.
3. Remove the baking sheet from the oven and immediately cover it tightly with aluminum foil. Set aside for 30 minutes, or until the peppers are cool enough to handle.
4. Remove the stem from each pepper and cut them into quarters. Remove the peels and seeds and place the peppers in a food processor, along with any juices that have collected. Discard the stems, peels, and seeds. Pour 1 tablespoon of the oil over the peppers. Puree the roasted red peppers and set aside.
5. Heat the remaining 1 tablespoon oil in a heavy saucepan over medium heat. Add the onion and sauté until translucent, about 3 minutes. Add the garlic and sauté for 1 more minute. Add the pepper puree and cook until the edges bubble, then decrease the heat and simmer for 10 minutes.
6. Add the anchovy paste (which is optional, but it will thicken this sauce nicely).
7. Add the beef broth a little at a time so that the sauce isn't too thin. Simmer for 5 minutes.

8. Add the basil, season with salt and pepper, and simmer for at least 15 minutes. You may simmer for longer, depending on how thick you want the sauce.

NOTE

Use this in place of tomato sauce in any recipe (such as the pizza on page 235).

Chili Garlic Paste

Makes ½ cup

15 dried whole chiles, preferably a mixture of hot and mild
2 tablespoons extra virgin olive oil
2 garlic cloves, peeled
kosher salt

1. Put the chiles in a bowl and cover with boiling water and a small plate to keep them submerged. Soak for 30 minutes, or until soft. Drain the chiles and reserve some of the soaking water.
2. Clean each chile by removing the stem, then pulling or slitting the chile open. Do this over a sink since they will contain a lot of water. Scrape out most of the seeds, retaining some if you want a hotter paste.
3. Put the chiles and any seeds you might be using in a blender or food processor, along with the oil, garlic, and a generous amount of salt. Puree until smooth, adding a spoonful of soaking water at a time, until the consistency is a thick paste.
4. Use immediately or cool, cover tightly, and refrigerate.

NOTE

This is great as a rub for any meat, poultry, or fish dish—especially if you like things a little spicy.

Avocado Pesto

Serves 2

3 garlic cloves, peeled
1 avocado, peeled and pitted
¼ cup almonds, crushed
¼ cup pine nuts
¼ cup watercress
4 tablespoons (½ stick) salted grass-fed butter, melted and
    slightly cooled
¼ cup grated Parmesan cheese
½ teaspoon freshly squeezed lemon juice

Combine the garlic and avocado in a food processor and process
until creamy. Add the remaining ingredients and pulse until
combined and the texture is to your liking.

NOTE
This pesto is great to serve on Parmesan crisps (page 177),
over shirataki noodles, or with spaghetti squash.

Traditional Pesto

Makes 1 cup

2 cups fresh basil leaves
½ cup pine nuts, toasted
1 cup grated Parmesan cheese
4 garlic cloves, peeled
¾ cup extra virgin olive oil
coarse sea salt and freshly ground black pepper
grated zest and juice of 1 lemon

Combine the basil, pine nuts, cheese, and garlic in a food processor
and pulse to combine. With the machine running, add the oil in
a slow, steady stream until well combined. Season with salt and

pepper, then stir in the lemon zest and juice. (If you won't be using the pesto right away, cover and refrigerate it before adding the lemon zest and juice. Stir them in just before serving.)

NOTE ··

Pesto goes great tossed with zucchini "noodles" or as a pizza topping.

Garlicky Tahini Sauce

Makes 1 cup

⅓ cup tahini
3 tablespoons freshly squeezed lemon juice
2 garlic cloves, minced
generous pinch red pepper flakes
⅓ cup water
coarse sea salt and freshly ground black pepper

In a medium bowl, stir together the tahini, lemon juice, garlic, and red pepper flakes. Whisk in the water until you have a smooth, blended sauce. Season generously with salt and black pepper.

NOTE ··

Try this over a lamb dish or any steamed vegetable to give the dish a more exotic flair.

Beverages and Desserts

I think sweet treats should be kept to a minimum or used for special occasions. But I thought you might enjoy a few to serve to guests.

Sweet Custard Pie

Serves 8

FOR THE CRUST

8 ounces macadamia nuts, ground
¼ cup lo han
¼ teaspoon coarse sea salt
4 tablespoons (½ stick) salted grass-fed butter, melted

FOR THE CUSTARD

3 large eggs or 6 large egg yolks
2 cups heavy cream
½ cup lo han or stevia
1 teaspoon pure vanilla extract
¼ teaspoon coarse sea salt

1. Preheat the oven to 325°F.
2. To make the crust, in a medium bowl combine the nuts, lo han, and salt. Add the melted butter and stir to combine.
3. Press the mixture into the bottom of a 9- or 10-inch cake, pie, or springform pan and set aside.
4. To make the custard, in a medium bowl, beat the eggs slightly, then add the cream, lo han, vanilla, and salt and stir well.
5. Pour the custard into the pie shell and bake until the custard is firm, about 30 minutes. Serve warm or chilled—it will almost be like two different desserts.

Chocolate-Coconut Pudding

Serves 2

1 avocado, pitted and peeled
1 cup unsweetened coconut milk
2 tablespoons unsweetened cocoa powder
2 tablespoons chia seeds

1. In a medium bowl, mash the avocado until very smooth. Stir in the milk and cocoa powder.
2. Divide the pudding evenly between two dessert bowls. Stir 1 tablespoon chia seeds into each, cover, and allow to set in the refrigerator for 2 hours or overnight. Serve chilled.

Guava Crème Brûlée

Serves 6

8 large egg yolks
1 cup heavy cream
1 cup frozen guava puree, thawed

1. Preheat the oven to 300°F. Place a kettle of water over high heat and bring to a boil.
2. Put the egg yolks in a mixing bowl and set aside.
3. In a small saucepan, bring the cream to a simmer over medium heat. As soon as it begins to simmer, remove the pan from the heat. Whisk the egg yolks vigorously while adding the cream in a slow, thin stream. Do not add the cream too quickly or the mixture will curdle.
4. Pour the cream mixture through a fine-mesh sieve into a bowl. Add the guava puree and stir until well blended.
5. Pour the mixture into six ½-cup ramekins and place them in a small baking dish. Carefully add boiling water to the baking dish to come halfway up the sides of the ramekins. Bake until set, about 45 minutes. Remove the ramekins from the water and set aside on a rack to cool.
6. Just prior to serving, scorch the top layer of the crème mixture under the broiler or with a handheld kitchen torch until lightly golden (you don't need sugar). Serve.

Chocolate Pudding

Serves 2

1 avocado, pitted and peeled
2 tablespoons unsweetened cocoa powder
SweetLeaf Liquid Stevia Sweet Drops, chocolate flavor

In a medium bowl, mash the avocado until smooth. Stir in the cocoa powder. Add stevia to taste and serve.

Chocolate–Peanut Butter Pudding

Serves 2

¼ cup chia seeds
1 teaspoon pure vanilla extract
1 cup unsweetened almond milk
2 scoops unsweetened chocolate protein powder
2 tablespoons peanut butter powder
2 tablespoons unsweetened cocoa powder
dash ground cinnamon
1 tablespoon unsweetened peanut butter

1. In a medium bowl, combine the chia seeds, vanilla extract, and almond milk. Slowly add the protein powder, peanut butter powder, cocoa powder, and cinnamon, whisking as you go. Protein and cocoa tend to clump, so whisk vigorously enough and long enough to make a smooth mixture.
2. Divide into two bowls and refrigerate for 15 minutes, allowing the mixture to thicken.
3. Prior to serving, top each bowl with half the peanut butter.

Peanut Butter Chocolate Chip Cookies

Makes 12 to 18

macadamia nut oil spray
1 cup unsweetened creamy or chunky peanut butter
¾ cup lo han
1 large egg, beaten
1 teaspoon baking soda
1 teaspoon pure vanilla extract
1 cup unsweetened chocolate chips

1. Preheat the oven to 350°F. Lightly coat a baking sheet with macadamia nut oil spray.
2. In a large bowl, combine all the ingredients and mix well.
3. Dollop a generous 1 tablespoon of the mixture for each cookie onto the prepared baking sheet, spacing them about an inch apart.
4. Bake until browned or your desired crispness, 10 to 20 minutes. Transfer the cookies to a wire rack to cool before serving.

Chocolate Milk

Serves 1

1 scoop CocoaLogic
1 cup unsweetened almond milk

Combine the CocoaLogic and milk in a glass and stir. Serve.

Chocolate Milkshake

Serves 1

1 scoop CocoaLogic
1 scoop unsweetened whey protein powder
1 tablespoon macadamia nut oil
¼ cup unsweetened cashew milk
ice

Combine all the ingredients in a blender and mix on high until thick, creamy, and decadent. Serve.

Mochaccino

Serves 1

1 scoop CocoaLogic
1 cup brewed coffee
ice

Combine all the ingredients in a blender and mix on high to your desired consistency. Serve.

CHAPTER TWELVE

The A-List Diet
30-Day Meal Plans

C learly you are not going to like *everything* that I include in this thirty-day plan. It is meant simply to be used as a guideline. I want you to get the idea of how to alkalinize your meals and vary your amino acids to maximize weight loss.

These suggested menus include only the three major meals (breakfast, lunch, and dinner). But don't forget, you also need your AM and PM protein boost shots and your daily protein booster shake for your dieting type. You can even make the protein booster shake one of your meals or a snack if you choose. I also did not include snacks or desserts, since those should be rare when you are on the A-list path to success. (But, as you can see, there are recipes for desserts, should you feel the urge; as for snacks, simply choose anything from the lists of foods you can have in unlimited quantities in chapter 4.)

I encourage you to experiment with your own favorite recipes, too—and to try new ones. Here are a few hints to help you convert some of your favorite recipes into ones suitable for your new A-list way of life:

Instead of	Try this
bread	thin to medium sliced eggplant (just don't overcook it)
buns	portobello mushroom caps
taco shells	leafy greens
mashed potatoes	mashed cauliflower
pizza crust	mushroom or cauliflower crust
pasta	zucchini "noodles," shirataki noodles, or calamari shreds

Think outside the box when it comes to planning your meals. Just because you're used to eating certain foods at certain times of the day doesn't mean you can *only* eat them then. There's nothing wrong with having a salad for breakfast or bacon and eggs for dinner. In fact, it can mix things up nicely and keep you from getting bored—which is a huge part of sticking with any diet.

So, without further ado, here are some suggested menus to get you through your first month as an A-Lister.

DAY 1

Breakfast

Fried Egg and Bacon with Watercress (page 163)

Lunch

Vegetable Soup (page 180)

Dinner

Turkey Chili (page 184)

DAY 2

Breakfast

Bitter Greens, Grapefruit, and Avocado Salad (page 191)

Lunch

Pork Stir-Fry with Broccolini and Peppers (page 224)

Dinner

Chili-Glazed Chicken Drumsticks with Slaw (page 218)

DAY 3

Breakfast

Zucchini Pasta with Greens and Goat Cheese(page 238)

Lunch

Parmesan Crisps Topped with Bacon, Egg, Pistachios, and Parsley (page 177) with Avocado Pesto (page 268)

Dinner

Chinese Roast Pork (page 221) with Stir-Fried Bok Choy and Garlic (page 254)

DAY 4

Breakfast

Mexican Fried Eggs (page 164)

Lunch

Tuna Melt on Portobello with Broccoli Sprouts (page 207)

Dinner

Vegetable Lasagna (page 237)

DAY 5

Breakfast

Sicilian Breakfast
Salad (page 165)

Lunch

Sriracha Steak on Swamp
Cabbage (page 226)

Dinner

Halibut with Salsa
Fresca (page 246) with
Mustardy Asparagus
(page 255)

DAY 6

Breakfast

Protein Crêpes with
Turkey Sausage (page 166)

Lunch

Chinese-Style Sashimi
(page 241)

Dinner

Coconut Buffalo Curry
(page 230)

DAY 7

Breakfast

Duck Eggs with
Brussels Sprouts and
Pancetta (page 171)

Lunch

Chicken and
Avocado Salad with Lime
Mayonnaise (page 212)

Dinner

Spicy Roast Duck (page 220)
with Sautéed Collard
Greens (page 254)

DAY 8

Breakfast

Pizza with
Chia Seed Meatballs
and Red Pepper Sauce
(page 235)

Lunch

My Favorite Burger
(page 203)

Dinner

Almond Soup
with Lump Crab
(page 185)

DAY 9

Breakfast

Rainbow Chard
Frittata (page 168)

Lunch

Chinese-Style Chicken
with Cashews (page 212)

Dinner

Adobo Chicken
with Mushrooms
(page 210)

DAY 10

Breakfast

Kohlrabi Salad
with Vegetable Dressing
(page 192)

Lunch

Grilled Prawns with
Cauliflower Tabbouleh
(page 242)

Dinner

Broiled Bluefish with Herbs
(page 247) with Roasted
Broccolini (page 255)

DAY 11

Breakfast

Chicken Breakfast
Skillet (page 170)

Lunch

Broccoli and Bacon
Salad (page 193)

Dinner

Turkey Fajitas (page 221)

DAY 12

Breakfast

Turmeric
Cauliflower Bowl
(page 239)

Lunch

Salmon-Stuffed
Cabbage
(page 243)

Dinner

Orange Beef
and Broccoli
(page 225)

DAY 13

Breakfast

Egg Foo Young
with Oysters (page 172)

Lunch

Taco Burger
Wrap (page 205)

Dinner

Italian Roast
Pork (page 222) with Fried
Marinated Zucchini
(page 262)

DAY 14

Breakfast

Protein Crêpes with Lox
and Cream Cheese
(page 167)

Lunch

Tuscan Salad with
Arctic Char
(page 194)

Dinner

Crispy Lamb with Cumin
(page 231)

DAY 15

Breakfast

Shakshuka (page 173)

Lunch

Monkfish Curry (page 244)

Dinner

Crusted Pike with
Asparagus (page 248)

DAY 16

Breakfast

Pumpkin Protein
Pancakes (page 168)

Lunch

Kale Caesar
Salad (page 195)

Dinner

Alaska King Crab
Legs (page 248) with
Creamed Brussels Sprouts
with Pancetta (page 256)

DAY 17

Breakfast

Portobello Mushroom Topped with Scrambled Eggs (page 177)

Lunch

Creole Gumbo (page 181)

Dinner

Roasted Mustardy Chicken (page 219)

DAY 18

Breakfast

Raw Kale and Hemp Seed Salad (page 192)

Lunch

Tri-Tip Gruyère Melt (page 208)

Dinner

Razor Clams with Kielbasa (page 249)

DAY 19

Breakfast

Japanese Eggs with Radish (page 174)

Lunch

Spinach Salad with Pattypan Squash (page 196)

Dinner

Steak Fajitas over Portobello Mushroom Strips (page 228)

DAY 20

Breakfast

Garlic Soup with Mascarpone and Chives (page 180)

Lunch

Chopped Spinach Cobb Salad (page 197)

Dinner

Grilled Swordfish (page 250) with Garlicky Stir-Fried Chinese Long Beans (page 257)

DAY 21

Breakfast

Smoked Mackerel
Cakes (page 176)

Lunch

Fennel and Avocado
Salad (page 198)

Dinner

Moroccan Leg of
Lamb (page 232) with
Sugar Snap Peas with
Horseradish (page 257)

DAY 22

Breakfast

Spaghetti Squash,
Taleggio, and
Okra Frittata (page 170)

Lunch

The Astoria
Greek Salad (page 198)

Dinner

Pepper Rib Eye Steak with
Watercress and Purslane
(page 227) with Braised
Celery (page 258)

DAY 23

Breakfast

Asian Vegetable
Salad (page 193)

Lunch

Chicken Cordon
Bleu Wedge
Burger (page 205)

Dinner

Fresh Ham (page 223)
with Zucchini-Basil
Gratin (page 258)

DAY 24

Breakfast

Breakfast Tartlets (page 175)

Lunch

Creamy
Avocado-Broccoflower
Soup (page 182)

Dinner

Grilled Cashew
Chicken (page 211) with
Frisée and Radicchio
Salad with Mustard
Vinaigrette (page 199)

DAY 25

Breakfast

Chili, Garlic, and Basil Chicken over Shirataki Noodles (page 217)

Lunch

Mushroom and Chia Seed Turkey Burger on Eggplant (page 206)

Dinner

Sea Bass Stew (page 187)

DAY 26

Breakfast

Pistachio Smoked Salmon Rolls (page 241)

Lunch

Swiss Cauliflower-Emmentaler Soup (page 183)

Dinner

Mother's Brisket (page 229) with Green Bean Casserole (page 261)

DAY 27

Breakfast

Fried Egg and Gruyère on a Bed of Avocado (page 163)

Lunch

Pizza Siciliano with Sardines, Anchovy Paste, and Broccoli Sprouts (page 236)

Dinner

Chicken Ragout with Shirataki Noodles (page 217)

DAY 28

Breakfast

Chicken Pesto (page 216)

Lunch

Bacon and Blue Cheese Stuffed Burger (page 204)

Dinner

Baked Salmon with Braised Fennel (page 251)

DAY 29

Breakfast

Parmesan Crisps Topped
with Bacon, Egg, Pistachios,
and Parsley (page 177)

Lunch

Avocado Salad with Alfalfa
Sprouts (page 199)

Dinner

Roast Leg of Veal with
Sausage Stuffing (page
233) with Whole Roasted
Cauliflower with Green
Herb Sauce (page 259)

DAY 30

Breakfast

Avocado Smoothie
(page 178)

Lunch

Parsley Gazpacho
(page 183)

Dinner

Stuffed Chicken with
Squash Ribbons
(page 214)

Resources

Go to AListDietBook.com for products, tips, and tricks to making the A-List Diet even easier.

You can also follow me on Twitter @alistdiet and on Facebook at A-List Diet Book.

To get my free e-letter Reality Health Check and other health news, go to DrPescatore.com.

I also recommend you check out the following websites, which are full of helpful information:

- LocalHarvest.org: Search for farms, farmers' markets, and CSAs near you.
- FoodSubs.com: Learn how to change up your favorite recipes easily.
- LowCarbontheTown.com: Find low-carb options at your favorite restaurants.
- LocalCatch.org: You can search by region to find your own community-supported fishery.
- OA.org: Get the support you need from Overeaters Anonymous.

Bibliography

CHAPTER 1

Academy of Nutrition and Dietetics. "The pH Miracle for Weight Loss Book Review." Retrieved August 10, 2012. http://www.eatrightpro.org/resource/media/trends-and-reviews/book-reviews/the-ph-miracle-for-weight-loss.

Adeva, M.M., et al. "Insulin Resistance and the Metabolism of Branched-Chain Amino Acids in Humans." *Amino Acids* 43, no. 1 (Jul. 2012): pp. 171–81.

"Alkaline Diets and Cancer: Fact or Fiction?" *Intelihealth*. https://web.archive.org/web/20150327162238/http://www.intelihealth.com/article/alkaline-diets-and-cancer-fact-or-fiction?.

Austel, A., et al. "Weight Loss with a Modified Mediterranean-Type Diet Using Fat Modification: A Randomized Controlled Trial." *European Journal of Clinical Nutrition* 69, no. 8 (2015): pp. 878–84. doi:10.1038/ejcn.2015.11.

Binder, E., et al. "Leucine Supplementation Protects from Insulin Resistance by Regulating Adiposity Levels." *PLOS ONE* 8, no. 9 (25 Sept. 2013): p. e74705. doi: 10.1371/journal.pone.0074705.

Canadian Cancer Society. "An Alkaline Diet and Cancer." Retrieved August 10, 2012. http://www.cancer.ca/en/prevention-and-screening/be-aware/cancer-myths-and-controversies/an-alkaline-diet-and-cancer/?region=on.

Candler, N., et al. "Effects of Prolonged Administration of Branched-Chain Amino Acids on Body Composition and Physical Fitness." *Minerva Endocrinologia* 20, no. 4 (Dec. 1995): pp. 217–23.

Cassileth, C.R. *Principles and Practice of Gastrointestinal Oncology.* Philadelphia, PA: Lippincott Williams & Wilkins, 2008: p. 137.

Cunningham, E. "What Impact Does pH Have on Food and Nutrition?" *Journal of the American Dietetic Association* 109, no. 10 (Oct. 2009): p. 1816. doi: 10.1016/j.jada.2009.08.028. PMID 19782182.

DAK-Studie, "Immer mehr Senioren mit Mangelernährung in Klinik." *Hamburger Abendblatt* (Dec. 2011).

Erdmann, R., et al. *The Amino Revolution*. New York: Touchstone, 1987.

Escott-Stump S., ed. *Nutrition and Diagnosis-Related Care*. 6th ed. Philadelphia, PA: Lippincott Williams & Wilkins, 2008.

Fenton, T.R., et al. "Causal Assessment of Dietary Acid Load and Bone Disease: A Systematic Review & Meta-Analysis Applying Hill's Epidemiologic Criteria for Causality." *Nutrition Journal* 10, no. 41 (2011). doi: 10.1186/1475-2891-10-41. PMC 3114717. PMID 21529374.

Fenton, T.R., et al. "Meta-Analysis of the Effect of the Acid-Ash Hypothesis of Osteoporosis on Calcium Balance." *Journal of Bone and Mineral Research* 11 (Nov. 2009): pp. 1835–40. doi:10.1359/jbmr.090515. PMID 19419322.

Fenton, T.R., et al. "Phosphate Decreases Urine Calcium and Increases Calcium Balance: A Meta-Analysis of the Osteoporosis Acid-Ash Diet Hypothesis." *Nutrition Journal* 8, no. 41 (2009). doi:10.1186/1475-2891-8-41. PMC 2761938. PMID 19754972.

Fogarty, A.W., et al. "A Prospective Study of Weight Change and Systemic Inflammation Over 9 Years." *American Journal of Clinical Nutrition* 87, no. 1 (Jan. 2008): pp. 30–35.

Food and Nutrition Board, Institute of Medicine of the National Academies. *Dietary Reference Intakes for Water, Potassium, Sodium, Chloride, and Sulfate*. Washington, D.C.: The National Academies Press, 2005: p. 189.

Food and Nutrition Board, Institute of Medicine, National Academies Press. "Dietary Reference Intakes for Energy, Carbohydrate, Fiber, Fat, Fatty Acids, Cholesterol, Protein and Amino Acids." *Journal of the American Dietetic Association* 102, no. 11 (2002): pp. 1621–30. doi: 10.17226/10490.

Jankovic, N., et al. "Adherence to a Healthy Diet According to the World Health Organization Guidelines and All-Cause Mortality in Elderly Adults From Europe and the United States." *American Journal of Epidemiology* 180, no. 10 (2014): pp. 978–88. doi: 10.1093/aje/kwu229.

Jitomir, J., et al. "Leucine For Retention of Lean Mass on a Hypo Caloric Diet." *Journal of Medicinal Food* 11, no. 4 (Dec. 2008): pp. 606–9.

Lasa, A., et al. "Comparative Effect of Two Mediterranean Diets Versus a Low-Fat Diet on Glycaemic Control in Individuals with Type 2 Diabetes." *European Journal of Clinical Nutrition* 68, no. 7 (2014): pp. 767–72. doi: 10.1038/ejcn.2014.1.

Laviano, A., et al. "Glutamine Supplementation Favors Weight Loss in Nondieting Obese Female Patients: A Pilot Study." *European Journal of Clinical Nutrition* 68, no. 11 (Nov. 2014): pp. 1264–66.

Layman, D.K., et al. "Potential Importance of Leucine in Treatment of Obesity and the Metabolic Syndrome." *Journal of Nutrition* 136 (Jan. 2006): pp. 319–23.

Mansour, A., et al. "Effect of Glutamine Supplementation on Cardiovascular Risk Factors in Patients with Type 2 Diabetes." *Nutrition* 31, no. 1 (Jan. 2015): pp. 119–26.

Mourier, A., et al. "Combined Effects of Caloric Restriction and Branched Chain Amino Acid Supplementation on Body Composition and Exercise Performance in Elite Wrestlers." *International Journal of Sports Medicine* 18, no. 1 (Jan. 1997): pp. 47–55.

National Center for Health Statistics, Centers for Disease Control and Prevention. "Leading Causes of Death." 2011: http://www.cdc.gov/NCHS/ fastats/Default.htm.

Nishimura, J., et al. "Isoleucine Prevents the Accumulation of Tissue Triglycerides and Up Regulates the Expression of PPARalpha and Uncoupling Protein in Diet-Induced Obese Mice." *Journal of Nutrition* 140, no. 3 (Mar. 2010): pp. 496–500.

Odo, S., et al. "A Pilot Clinical Trial on L-Carnitine Supplementation in Combination with Motivation Training: Effects on Weight Management in Healthy Volunteers." *Food and Nutrition Sciences* 4, no. 2 (2013): pp. 222–31. doi: 10.4236/fns.2013.42030.

Prada, P.O., et al. "L-glutamine Supplementation Induces Insulin Resistance in Adipose Tissue and Improves Insulin Signaling in Liver and Muscle with Diet-Induced Obesity." *Diabetologia* 50, no. 9 (2007): pp. 149–59.

Qin, L.Q., et al. "Higher Branched-Chain Amino Acid Intake is Associated with a Lower Prevalence of Being Overweight or Obese in Middle-Aged East Asian and Western Adults." *Journal of Nutrition* 141, no. 2 (Feb. 2011): pp. 249–54.

Remer, T., "Influence of Diet on Acid-Base Balance." *Seminars in Dialysis* 13, no. 4 (2000). doi:10.1046/j.1525-139x.2000.00062.x. PMID 10923348.

Shah, SH., et al. "Branched-Chain Amino Acid Levels Are Associated with Improvement in Insulin Resistance with Weight Loss." *Diabetologia* 55, no. 2 (Feb. 2012): pp. 321–30.

Williams, Sue. *Basic Nutrition and Diet Therapy*. 11th ed. St. Louis, MO: Mosby, 2001: p. 414.

Wutzke, KD., et al. "The Effect of L-Carnitine on Fat Oxidation, Protein Turnover, and Body Composition in Slightly Overweight Subjects." *Metabolism* 53, no. 8 (Aug. 2004): pp. 1002–6.

Zhang, J.J., et al. "L-Carnitine Ameliorated Fasting-Induced Fatigue, Hunger, and Metabolic Abnormalities in Patients With Metabolic Syndrome: A Randomized Controlled Study." *Nutrition Journal* 13 (26 Nov. 2014): p. 110.

CHAPTER 2

"Effect of Hormone Replacement Therapy on Cardiovascular Events in Recently Postmenopausal Women: Randomised Trial." *BMJ* (9 October 2012): p. 345.

"Impact of Insufficient Sleep on Total Daily Energy Expenditure, Food Intake, and Weight Gain." *Proceedings of the National Academy of Sciences of the United States of America* (11 Mar. 2013).

CHAPTER 3

Féher, J., et al. "Silymarin in the Prevention and Treatment of Liver Diseases and Primary Liver Cancer." *Current Pharmaceutical Biotechnology* 13, no. 1 (Jan. 2012): pp. 210–7.

Georgiou, G. "Natural Heavy Metal Chelators: Do They Work?" *Explore!* 16, no. 6 (2007).

Head, K.A. "Natural Approaches to Prevention and Treatment of Infections of the Lower Urinary Tract." *Alternative Medicine Review* 13, no. 3 (Sep. 2008): pp. 227–44.

Hun, L. "Bacillus Coagulans Significantly Improved Abdominal Pain and Bloating in Patients With IBS." *Postgraduate Medical Journal* 121, no. 2 (Mar. 2009): pp. 119–24.

Kidd, P., et al. "A Review of the Bioavailability and Clinical Efficacy of Milk Thistle Phytosome: A Silybin-Phosphatidylcholine Complex (Siliphos)." *Alternative Medicine Review* 10, no. 3 (Sep. 2005): pp. 193–203.

Nuttall, SL., et al. "An Evaluation of the Antioxidant Activity of a Standardized Grape Seed Extract, Leucoselect." *Journal of Clinical Pharmacy and Therapeutics* 23, no. 5 (1998) pp. 385–9.

Sharma, O.P. "Antioxidant Activity of Curcumin and Related Compounds." *Biochemistry Pharmacology* 25, no. 15 (1976): pp. 1811–12.

Tokaç, M., et al. "Protective Effects of Curcumin against Oxidative Stress Parameters and DNA Damage in the Livers and Kidneys of Rats with Biliary Obstruction." *Food and Chemistry Toxicology* (29 Jan. 2013).

Watson, N.F., et al. "Sleep Duration and Body Mass Index in Twins: A Gene-Environment Interaction." *Sleep Research Society Foundation, SLEEP* 35, no. 5 (2012): pp. 597–603.

Yarnell, E. "Botanical Medicines for the Urinary Tract." *World Journal of Urology* 20, no. 5 (Nov. 2002): 285–93.

CHAPTER 5

Afzal, S., et al. "Low Vitamin D and Hypertension: A Causal Association?" *Lancet* (25 Jun. 2014).

Aguilar, M., et al. "Prevalence of the Metabolic Syndrome in the United States, 2003–2012." *JAMA* 313, no. 19 (19 May 2015).

Andujar, I., et al. "Cocoa Polyphenols and Their Potential Benefits for Human Health." *Oxidative Medicine and Cellular Longevity* Volume 2012 (2012), Article ID 906252, 23 pages. http://dx.doi.org/10.1155/2012/906252.

Arwert, L.I., et al. "Effects of an Oral Mixture Containing Glycine, Glutamine, and Niacin on Memory, GH and IGF-I Secretion in Middle-Aged and Elderly Subjects." *Nutritional Neuroscience* 6, no. 5 (November 2003):269-75.

Barona, J., et al. "Grape Polyphenols Reduce Blood Pressure and Increase Flow-Mediated Vasodilation in Men with Metabolic Syndrome." *Journal of Nutrition* 142, no. 9 (Sep. 2012): pp. 1626–32. doi: 10.3945/jn.112.162743. Epub 2012 Jul 18.

Beauman, J.G. "Genital herpes: a review." *Am Fam Physician* 2005 72, no. 8 (Oct. 2005): pp. 1527–34.

Belcaro, G., et al. "Antioxidant Activity, Weight Management: GreenSelect® Phytosome® Green Tea Extract." *Evid Based Complement Alternat Med* 2013, Art. 869061 (2013).

Belcaro, G., et al. "French Oak Wood (Quercus robur) Extract (Robuvit®) in Primary Lymphedema: A Supplement, Pilot, Registry Evaluation." *International Journal of Angiology* 24, no. 1 (Mar. 2015): pp. 47–54. Published online 2014 Dec 15. doi: 10.1055/s-0034-1395982.

Belcaro, G., et al. "French Oak Wood Extract (Robuvit®) Reduces the Wheal and Flare Response to Histamine and Decreases Capillary Filtration in Normal Subjects." *Minerva Biotecnologica* 25, no. 4 (2013): pp. 199–205.

Belcaro, G., et al. "Improved Management of Primary Chronic Fatigue Syndrome with the Supplement French Oak Wood Extract (Robuvit®): A Pilot, Registry Evaluation." *Panminerva Medica* 56, no. 1 (2014): pp. 63–72.

Belcaro, G., et al. "Improvement of Common Cold with Pycnogenol®: A Winter Registry Study." *Panminerva Medica* 56, no. 4 (2014): pp. 301–8.

Belcaro, G., et al. "Pycnogenol® Improves Cognitive Function, Attention, Mental Performance, and Specific Professional Skills in Healthy Professionals Aged 35–55." *Journal of Neurosurgical Sciences* 58, no. 4 (2014): pp. 239–48.

Belcaro, G., et al. "Pycnogenol® Supplementation Improves Health Risk Factors in Subjects with Metabolic Syndrome." *Phytotherapy Research* 27, no. 10 (Oct. 2013): pp. 1572–8. doi: 10.1002/ptr.4883. Epub 2013 Jan 28.

Belcaro, G., et al. "Robuvit® (French Oak Wood Extract) in the Management of Functional, Temporary Hepatic Damage. A Registry, Pilot Study." *Minerva Medica* 105, no. 1 (2014): pp. 41–50.

Belcaro, G., et al. "Robuvit® (Quercus Robur Extract) Supplementation in Subjects With Chronic Fatigue Syndrome and Increased Oxidative Stress." *A Pilot Registry Study J Neurosurg Sci* 59 (2015): pp. 105–17.

Bellon, G., et al. "Glutamine Increases Collagen Gene Transcription in Cultured Human Fibroblasts." *Biochimica et Biophysica Acta* 1268, no. 3 (Sep. 1995): pp. 311–23.

Bendix, L., et al. "Association of Leukocyte Telomere Length with Fatigue in Nondisabled Older Adults." *Journal of Aging Research* Volume 2014 (2014), Article ID 403253, 8 pages, http://dx.doi.org/10.1155/2014/403253.

Breau, R.H., et al. "The effects of lysine anaolgs during pelvic surgery: a systematic review and meta-analysis." *Transfus Med Rev.* 28, no. 3 (2014): pp. 145–55.

Brickman, A.M., et al. "Enhancing Dentate Gyrus Function with Dietary Flavanols Improves Cognition in Older Adults." *Nature Neuroscience* Volume 17, 1798–1803 (2014) doi:10.1038/nn.3850.

Chuengsamarn, S., et al. "Curcumin Extract for Prevention of Type 2 Diabetes." *Diabetes Care* 35, no. 11 (2012): pp. 2121–27.

Cocchi, R. "Antidepressive Properties of L-glutamine: Preliminary Report." *Acta Psychologica Belgica* 76 (1976): pp. 658–66.

Cooper, AJ. "Role of Glutamine in Cerebral Nitrogen Metabolism and Ammonia Neurotoxicity." *Mental Retardation and Developmental Disabilities Research Reviews* 7, no. 4 (2001): pp. 280–6.

Corpus, E., et al. "Human Growth Hormone and Human Aging." *Endocrine Reviews* 299, no. 1 (11 Jul. 2008): pp. 64–71.

Crozier, S.J., et al. "Cacao Seeds Are a "Super Fruit": A Comparative Analysis of Various Fruit Powders and Products." *Chemistry Central Journal* 20115:5 doi: 10.1186/1752-153X-5-5.

Daniells, S. "Magnesium May Benefit Blood Pressure in Hypertensives." Nutraingredients.com (19 May 2009).

Deakova, Z., et al. "Influence of Oak Wood Polyphenols on Cysteine, Homocysteine, and Glutathione Total Levels and PON1 Activities in Human Adult Volunteers: A Pilot Study." *General Physiology and Biophysics* 34, no. 1 (2015): pp. 73–80.

Detopoulou, P., et al. "Dietary Antioxidant Capacity and Concentration of Adiponectin in Apparently Healthy Adults: The ATTICA Study." *European Journal of Clinical Nutrition* 64, no. 2 (2009): pp. 161–68.

Dietary Guidelines for Americans. Rockville, MD: U.S. Department of Health and Human Services and U.S. Department of Agriculture; 2005.

DiNicolantonio, J.J., et al. "L-Carnitine in the Secondary Prevention of Cardiovascular Disease: Systematic Review and Meta-Analysis." *Mayo Clinical Proceedings* 88, no. 6 (June 2013): pp. 544–51.

Di Pierro, F., et al. "GreenSelect® Phytosome as an Adjunct to a Low-Calorie Diet for Treatment of Obesity: A Clinical Trial." *Alternative Medicine Review* 14, no. 2 (2009).

"Do Multivitamins Work? Jury Is Still Out, but New Research Says No." news.com.au, video published 18 December 2013. http://www.news.com.au/lifestyle/health/do-multivitamins-work-jury-is-still-out-but-new-research-says-no/news-story/8ec61b1cec2e4ac98272e6bbccc6ec93.

Eathakkattu, A.B.S., et al. "Cross-Sectional and Longitudinal Associations between Circulating Leptin and Knee Cartilage Thickness in Older Adults." *Annual of the Rheumatic Diseases* 74, no. 1 (2015): pp. 82–88.

Ellam, S., et al. "Cacao and Human Health." *Annual Review of Nutrition* 33 (2013): pp. 105–28.

Faridi, Z., et al. "Acute Dark Chocolate and Cocoa Ingestion and Endothelial Function: A Randomized Controlled Crossover Trial." *The American Journal of Clinical Nutrition* 88, no. 1 (Jul. 2008): 58–63.

Fini, M., et al. "Effect of L-lysine and L-arginine osteoblast cultures from normal and osteopenic rats." *Biomed Pharmacother* 55, no. 4 (2001): pp. 213–20.

Forester, S.C., et al. "Inhibition of Starch Digestion by the Green Tea Polyphenol, (-)-Epigallocatechin-3-Gallate." *Molecular Nutrition & Food Research* 56, no. 11 (2012): pp. 1647–54.

Gaby, A.R. "Natural Remedies for Herpes Simplex." *Altern Med Rev* 11, no. 2 (Jun. 2006): 93–101.

Gad, M.Z. "Anti-Aging Effects of L-Arginine." *Journal of Advanced Research* 1, no. 3 (2010).

Garcia, R., et al. "Blood Amino Acids Concentration During Insulin Induced Hypoglycemia in Rats: The Role of Alanine and Glutamine in Glucose Recovery." *Amino Acids* 33, no. 1 (Jul. 2007).

Ghorbani, Z., et al. "Anti-Hyperglycemic and Insulin Sensitizer Effects of Turmeric and Its Principle Constituent Curcumin." *International Journal of Endocrinology and Metabolism* 12, no. 4 (2014).

Hassett, A.L., et al. "Pain Is Associated with Short Leukocyte Telomere Length in Women with Bromyalgia." *Journal of Pain* 13, no. 10 (2012): pp. 959–69.

Haytowitz, D.B., et al. "USDA Database for the Oxygen Radical Absorbance Capacity (ORAC) of Selected Foods, Release 2." *U.S. Department of Agriculture* (2010). http://www.orac-info-portal.de/download/ORAC_R2.pdf.

Herrera-Cordero, I., et al. "Cocoa Flavonoids Improve Insulin Signalling and Modulate Glucose Production via AKT and AMPK in HepG2 Cells." *Molecular Nutrition and Food Research* 57, no. 6 (Jun. 2013): pp. 974–85.

Higdon, J. "Resveratrol." Linus Pauling Institute, Oregon State University (2005). http://lpi.oregonstate.edu/mic/dietary-factors/phytochemicals/resveratrol.

Hussein, G., et al. "Astaxanthin Ameliorates Features of Metabolic Syndrome." *Life Sciences* 80, no. 6 (2007): pp. 522–29.

Indena. "Meriva®." http://www.meriva.info/en/meriva-bioavailable-curcumin/scientific-support/#bibliography.

"Insomnia." NIH Senior Health, last reviewed December 2012. https://nihseniorhealth.gov/sleepandaging/insomnia/01.html.

Iuorno, M.J., et al. "Effects of d-chiro-inositol in Lean Women with the Polycystic Ovary Syndrome." *Endocrine Practice* 2002 Nov-Dec;8(6):417-23.

Karna, E., et al. "The Potential Mechanism for Glutamine-Induced Collagen Biosynthesis in Cultured Human Skin Fibroblasts." *Comparative Biochemistry and Physiology* 130, no. 1 (Aug. 2001): pp. 23–32.

Kidd, P. "Astaxanthin, Cell Membrane Nutrient with Diverse Clinical Benefits and Anti-Aging Potential." *Alternative Medicine Review* 16, no. 4 (2011): pp. 355–64.

Kimanthi, K. "Farmer Finds Lucrative Tea Market in the East." *Daily Nation* (13 Feb. 2015).

Kohama, T., et al. "Effect of Low-dose French Maritime Pine Bark Extract on Climacteric Syndrome in 170 Perimenopausal Women: A Randomized, Double-Blind, Placebo-Controlled Trial." *The Journal of Reproductive Medicine* 58, no. 1–2 (Jan.–Feb. 2013): pp. 39–46.

Krymchantowski, A.V., et al. "Oral lysine clonixinate in the acute treatment of migraine: a double-blind placebo-controlled study." *Arq Neuropsiquiatr* 59, no. 1 (2001): pp. 46–49.

Kumar, A., et al. "Molecular Vibrations and Normal Modes in L-prolyl-glycyl-glycine Using Wilson GF Matrix Method." *Indian Journal of Biochemistry & Biophysics* 44 (Dec. 2007): pp. 450–7.

Le Chatelier, E., et al. "Richness of Human Gut Microbiome Correlates with Metabolic Markers." *Nature* (29 Aug. 2013): pp. 541–46.

Lee, B.J., et al. "A Significant Correlation between the Plasma Levels of Coenzyme Q10 and Vitamin B-6 and a Reduced Risk of Coronary Artery Disease." *Nutrition Research* 32, no. 10 (2012): pp. 751–56.

Lee, J., et al. "Telomerase Deficiency Affects Normal Brain Functions in Mice." *Neurochemical Research* 35, no. 2 (2010): pp. 211–18.

Lee, S., et al. "Effects of Oral Magnesium Supplementation on Insulin Sensitivity and Blood Pressure in Normo-Magnesemic Nondiabetic Overweight Korean Adults." *Nutrition, Metabolism, and Cardiovascular Diseases* 19 (2009): pp. 781–8.

Lieb, G. "Metabolic Syndrome on the Rise in America." *Pioneer News* (20 May 2015).

Liu, Y., et al. "Effect of Resveratrol on Blood Pressure: A Meta-Analysis of Randomized Controlled Trials." *Clinical Nutrition* 34, no. 1 (2015): pp. 27–34.

Luzzi, R., et al. "Improvement in Symptoms and Cochlear Flow with Pycnogenol® in Patients with Meniere's Disease and Tinnitus." *Minerva Medica* 105, no. 3 (2014): pp. 245–54.

Massolt, E.T., et al. "Appetite Suppression through Smelling of Dark Chocolate Correlates with Changes in Ghrelin in Young Women." *Regulatory Peptides* 161, no. 1–3 (9 Apr. 2010): pp. 81–6.

Mastroiacovo, D., et al. "Cocoa Flavanol Consumption Improves Cognitive Function, Blood Pressure Control, and Metabolic Profile in Elderly Subjects: The Cocoa, Cognition, and Aging (CoCoA) Study—A

Randomized Controlled Trial." *American Journal of Clinical Nutrition* (2014). December 17, 2014, doi: 10.3945/ajcn.114.092189.

McKay, J.A., et al. "Diet Induced Epigenetic Changes and Their Implications for Health." *Acta Physiologica* 202, no. 2 (2011): pp. 103–18.

Miyake, M., et al. "Randomised Controlled Trial of the Effects of L-Ornithine on Stress Markers and Sleep Quality in Healthy Workers." *Nutrition Journal* (2014).13:53. doi: 10.1186/1475-2891-13-53.

Morimoto, C., et al. "Anti-Obese Action of Raspberry Ketone." *Life Sciences* 77, no. 2 (May): pp. 194–204.

Murakami, H., et al. "Importance of Amino Acid Composition to Improve Skin Collagen Protein Synthesis Rates in UV-Irradiated Mice." *Amino Acids* 42, no. 6 (Jun. 2012): pp. 2481–9.

Neergaard, L. "Two New Studies Debunk Benefits of Multivitamins." NBCnews.com, video published 16 December 2013. http://www.nbcnews.com/health/two-new-studies-debunk-benefits-multivitamins-2D11757314.

Nehlig, A. "The Neuroprotective Effects of Cocoa Flavanol and Its Influence on Cognitive Performance." *British Journal of Clinical Pharmacology* (2012).

Nelson, F.R., et al. "The Effects of an Oral Preparation Containing Hyaluronic Acid (Oralvisc) on Obese Knee Osteoarthritis Patients Determined by Pain, Function, Bradykinin, Leptin, Inflammatory Cytokines, and Heavy Water Analyses." *Rheumatol International* 105 (2015): pp. 948–57.

"New Diet Lets You Eat Chocolate and Lose Weight." Pittsburgh.CBSlocal.com, video published 7 February 2014. http://pittsburgh.cbslocal.com/2014/02/07/new-diet-lets-you-eat-chocolate-and-lose-weight/

"Niacin (Vitamin B3, Nicotinic Acid), Niacinamide." *Mayo Clinic*, last updated 1 November 2013. http://www.mayoclinic.org/drugs-supplements/niacin--niacinamide/safety/hrb-20059838.

Nishida, Y., et al. "Quenching Activities of Common Hydrophilic and Lipophilic Antioxidants against Singlet Oxygen Using Chemiluminescence Detection System." *Carotenoid Science* 11 (2007): pp. 16–20.

Nishihira, J., et al. "The Discovery of a Novel Functional Constituent Extracted from Asparagus: Its Effectiveness for Stress Reduction, and Potential Use for Prevention of Sleep Disorders." Department of Medical Management and Informatics, Hokkaido Information University, Japan (unpublished, funded by Amino Up Chemical Co. Ltd.).

Orszachova, Z., et al. "An Effect of Oak-Wood Extract (Robuvit®) on Energy State of Healthy Adults-A Pilot Study." *Phytotherapy Research* 29, no. 8 (2015).

Otero, M., et al. "Towards a Pro-Inflammatory and Immunomodulatory Emerging Role of Leptin." *Rheumatology* 45, no. 8 (Aug. 2006): pp. 944–50.

Park, H.J., et al. "The Effects of Astragalus Membranaceus on Repeated Restraint Stress-Induced Biochemical and Behavioral Responses." *Korean Journal of Physiology and Pharmacology* 13, no. 4 (2009): pp. 315–19.

Park, K.S. "Raspberry Ketone Increases Both Lipolysis and Fatty Acid Oxidation in 3T3-L1 Adipocytes." *Planta Medica* 76, no. 15 (2010): pp. 1654–58.

Pase, M.P., et al. "Cocoa Polyphenols Enhance Positive Mood States but Not Cognitive Performance: A Randomized, Placebo-Controlled Trial." *Journal of Psychopharmacology* 27, no. 5 (May 2013): pp. 451–8.

Pietta P.G., et al. "Relationship Between Rate and Extent of Catechin Absorption and Plasma Antioxidant Status." *Biochem. Mol. Biol. Intl.* 46 (1998): pp. 895–903.

Prada, P.O., et al. "L-Glutamine Supplementation Induces Insulin Resistance in Adipose Tissue and Improves Insulin Signaling in Liver and Muscle of Rats with Diet-Induced Obesity." *Diabetologia* 50, no. 9 (2007).

Preidt, R. "Low Vitamin D Levels Linked to High Blood Pressure." *HealthDay News* (26 Jun. 2014).

"Purple Tea with GHG Overview." *Maypro.* http://maypro.com/sites/default/files/studies/Purple%20Tea%20with%20GHG.PDF.

Ramesh, V., et al. "Significant of Wine and Reseveratrol in Cardiovascular Disease: French Paradox Revisited." *Experimental and Clinical Cardiology* 11, no. 3 (2006): pp. 217–25.

Rao, M., et al. "Inhibition of Histone Lysine Methylation Enhances Cancer-Testis Antigen Expression in Lung Cancer Cells: Implications for Adoptive Immunotherapy of Cancer." *Cancer Res* 71, no. 12 (2011): p. 4129204.

Renaud, S. "Serge Renaud and the French Paradox: The Origin of Interest in Wine and Health." *The Prince of Pinot* 9, no. 19 (2013).

Renaud, S., et al. "Wine, Alcohol, Platelets, and the French Paradox for Coronary Heart Disease." *Lancet* 339, no. 8808 (20 Jun. 1992): pp. 1523–6.

"Robuvit® (Quercus Robur Extract) Supplementation in Subjects with Chronic Fatigue Syndrome and Increased Oxidative Stress: A Pilot Registry Study." *Journal of Neurosurgical Sciences* 59, no. 2 (2015): pp. 105–17.

Sanmukhani, J., et al. "Efficacy and Safety of Curcumin in Major Depressive Disorder." *Phytotherapy Research* 28, no. 4 (2014): pp. 579–85.

Simonetti P., et al. "Treatment of Chronic Hepatitis Using Whey Protein (non-heated)." *16th International Congress of Nutrition.* July/August, Montreal, Canada (1997).

Singh, B.B., et al. "Safety and Effectiveness of an L-Lysine, Zinc, and Herbal-Based Product on the Treatment of Facial and Circumoral Herpes." *Altern Med Rev* 10, no. 2 (2005): pp. 123–7.

Sivonova, M., et al. "The Effect of Pycnogenol® on the Erythrocyte Membrane Fluidity." *General Physiology Biophysics* 23, no. 1 (2004): pp. 39–51.

Sorond, F.A., et al. "Neurovascular Coupling, Cerebral White Matter Integrity, and Response to Cocoa in Older People." *Official Journal of the American Academy of Neurology* 81, no. 10 (3 Sep. 2013): pp. 904–9.

Stanislavov, R., et al. "Improvement of Erectile Function by a Combination of French Maritime Pine Bark and Roburins with Amino Acids." *Minerva Urologica e Nefrologica* 67, no. 1 (2015): pp. 27–32.

Stanislavov, R., et al. "Sperm Quality in Men Is Improved by Supplementation with a Combination of L-Arginine, L-Citrullin, Roburins and Pycnogenol®." *Minerva Urologica e Nefrologica* 66, no. 4 (2014): pp. 217–23.

Stechmiller, J. K., PhD, ARNP; Beverly Childress, MSN; Tricia Porter, BSN Arginine Immunonutrition in Critically Ill Patients: A Clinical Dilemma, *Am J Crit Care* 13, no. 1 (2004).

Tfelf-Hansen, P. "The Effectiveness of Combined Oral Lysine Acetylsalicylate and Metoclopramide in the Treatment of Migraine Attacks. Comparison with Placebo andOoral Sumatriptan." *Funct Neurol* 15, suppl. 3 (2000): pp. 196–201.

"The French Paradox." CBSnews.com (2009): http://www.cbsnews.com/videos/the-french-paradox/.

"Triglycerides More Important Than Cholesterol in Stroke Risk." Bupa, last updated 16 March 2011. https://www.bupa.com.au/health-and-wellness/health-information/heart-health/risks-and-prevention/risk-factors/doc/triglycerides-more-important-than-cholesterol-in-stroke-risk.

Vangsness, S. "Alkaline Diet." Nuts.com, published 16 January 2013.

"Vitamin B12." *WebMD.* http://www.webmd.com/vitamins-supplements/ingredientmono-926-vitamin%20b12.aspx?activeingredientid=926.

"Vitamin C (Ascorbic Acid)." *WebMD.* http://www.webmd.com/vitamins-supplements/ingredientmono-1001-vitamin%20c%20ascorbic%20acid.aspx?activeingredientid=1001.

"Vitamin D." *WebMD.* http://www.webmd.com/vitamins-supplements/ingredientmono-929-vitamin%20d.aspx?activeingredientid=929.

"Vitamin E." *WebMD.* http://www.webmd.com/vitamins-supplements/ingredientmono-954-vitamin%20e.aspx?activeingredientid=954.

"Wait, Multivitamins Don't Work?" *New York Post*, 17 December 2013.

Waki, H., et al. "Effect of Enzyme-Treated Asparagus (ETAS) on the Stress Response Substance in a Clinical Trial." *Clinical Nutrition* 32 (2013): pp. S233–S234.

Walton, A.G. "How Much Sugar Are Americans Eating?" *Forbes,* Aug. 2012.

Wang, L., et al. "Raspberry Ketone Protects Rats Red High-Fat Diets Against Nonalcoholic Steatohepatitis." *Journal of Medicinal Food* 15, no. 5 (2012): pp. 495–503.

Wax, E. "Riboflavin." *Medline Plus*, last modified 2 February 2, 2015. Web.

Wax, E. "Thiamin." *Medline Plus*, last modified 2 February 2, 2015. Web.

Welbourne, T.C. "Increased Plasma Bicarbonate and Growth Hormone after an Oral Glutamine Load." *The American Journal of Clinical Nutrition* (1995).

Winkler, G., et al. "Effectiveness of Different Benofotiamine Dosage Regimens in the Treatment of Painful Diabetic Neuropathy." *Thieme* (1999).

Yang, Y.S., et al. "Lipid-Lowering Effects of Curcumin in Patients with Metabolic Syndrome: A Randomized, Double-Blind, Placebo-Controlled Trial." *Phytotherapy Research* 28, no. 12 (2014).

CHAPTER 6

Albrecht, J., et al. "Roles of Glutamine in Neurotransmission." *Neuron Glia Biology* (2010).

Alexander, S. "Cheese: The Secret to a Longer Life and Faster Metabolism?" *The Telegraph* (Apr. 2015).

"Are Telomeres the Key to Aging and Cancer? Learn." Genetic Science Learning Center. Last updated 2014. Accessed November 2014.

Barbul, A., et al. "Arginine Enhances Wound Healing and Lymphocyte Immune Response in Humans." *Surgery* 108, no. 2 (1990): pp. 331–37.

Boelens, P.G., et al. "Glutamine Alimentation in Catabolic State." *The Journal of Nutrition* 131, no. 9 (1 Sep. 2001): pp. 2569S–2577S.

Brouilette, S.W., et al. "Telomere Length, Risk of Coronary Heart Disease, and Statin Treatment in the West of Scotland Primary Prevention Study: A Nested Case-Control Study." *Lancet* 396, no. 9556 (Jan. 13, 2007): pp. 107–14).

Crous-Bou, M., et al. "Mediterranean Diet and Telomere Length in Nurses' Health Study: Population Based Cohort Study." *BMJ* 349 (2014): p. g6674.

Demissie, S., et al. "Insulin Resistance, Oxidative Stress, Hypertension, and Leukocyte Telomere Length in Men from the Framingham Heart Study." *Aging Cell* 5, no. 4 (2006): pp. 325–30.

Desneves, K.J., et al. "Treatment with Supplementary Arginine, Vitamin C, and Zinc in Patients with Pressure Ulcers: A Randomized Controlled Trial." *Clinical Nutrition* 24, no. 6 (2005): pp. 979–87.

Gran, P., et al. "Muscle p70S6K Phosphorylation in Response to Soy and Dairy Rich Meals in Middle Aged Men with Metabolic Syndrome: A Randomized Crossover Trial." *Nutrition & Metabolism* 11 (2014): p. 46.

Hoffman, J.R., et al. "Examination of the Efficacy of Acute L-Alanyl-L-Glutamine Ingestion during Hydration Stress in Endurance Exercise." *Journal of the International Society of Sports Nutrition* 7 (3 Feb. 2010): p. 8. doi: 10.1186/1550-2783-7-8.

Huffman, F.G., et al. "L-Glutamine Supplementation Improves Nelfinavir-Associated Diarrhea in HIV-Infected Individuals." *HIV Clinical Trials* 4 (2003): pp. 324–9.

Koeth, R.A., et al. "Intestinal Microbiota Metabolism of L-Carnitine, a Nutrient in Red Meat, Promotes Atherosclerosis." *Nature Medicine* 19, no. 5 (2013): pp. 576–85.

Kuhn, K.S., et al. "Glutamine As Indispensible Nutrient in Oncology: Experimental and Clinical Evidence." *European Journal of Nutrition* 49, no. 4 (Jun. 2010): pp. 197–210.

Mansour, A., et al. "Effect of Glutamine Supplementation on Cardiovascular Risk Factors in Patients with Type 2 Diabetes." *Nutrition* 31, no. 1 (Jan. 2015): 119–26.

Prescott, B. "Glutamine Supplements Show Promise In Treating Stomach Ulcers." *Beth Israel Deaconess Medical Center* (2009). http://www.bidmc.org/News/PRLandingPage/2009/May/Stomach-Ulcers.aspx.

Rudakov, V.V., et al. "Effect of Low Doses of X-Ray Irradiation on the Nonspecific Protective Systems and the Gamma Globulin Concentration in the Blood of Chicks." *Radiobiologia* 18, no. 6 (1978): pp. 914–5.

Sampson, M.J., et al. "Monocyte Telomere Shortening and Oxidative DNA Damage in Type 2 Diabetes." *Diabetes Care* 29, no. 2 (2006): pp. 283–89.

Simpson, C.W., et al. "Glycyl-L-Glutamine Injected Centrally Suppresses Alcohol Drinking in P Rats." *Alcohol* 42, no. 2 (Mar. 2008): pp. 99–106.

"The 2009 Nobel Prize in Physiology or Medicine: Press Release." Nobelprize.org. Published October 5, 2009. Accessed November 10, 2014. https://www.nobelprize.org/nobel_prizes/medicine/laureates/2009/press.html.

Valdes, A.M., et al. "Telomere Length in Leukocytes Correlates with Bone Mineral Density and Is Shorter in Women with Osteoporosis." *Osteoporosis International* 18, vol. 9 (Sept. 2007): pp. 1203–10.

Van Anholt, R.D., et al. "Specific Nutritional Support Accelerates Pressure Ulcer Healing and Reduces Wound Care Intensity in Non-Malnourished Patients." *Nutrition* 26, no. 9 (2010): pp. 867–72.

Van der Harst, et al. "Telomere Length of Circulating Leukocytes Is Decreased in Patients with Chronic Heart Failure." *Journal of American College of Cardiology* 19, no. 13 (2007): pp. 1459-1464.

Van der Hulst, R.W.J., et al. "Glutamine and the Preservation of Gut Integrity." *Lancet* 341, no. 8857 (29 May 1993): pp. 1363–5.

CHAPTER 7

Adamson, I., et al. "A Supplement of Dikanut (Irvingia gabonesis) Improves Treatment of Type II Diabetics." *West African Journal of Medicine* 9, no. 2 (Apr.–Jun. 1990): pp. 108–15.

Baranski, M., et al. "Higher Antioxidant and Lower Cadmium Concentrations and Lower Incidence of Pesticide Residues in Organically Grown Crops: A Systematic Literature Review and Meta-Analyses." *British Journal of Nutrition* 112, no. 5 (14 Sept. 2014): pp. 794–811.

Bazzano, L.A., et al. "Effects of Low-Carbohydrate and Low-Fat Diets: A Randomized Trial." *Annals of Internal Medicine* 161, no. 5 (2014): pp. 309–318.

"Big Intake of High-Fat Dairy May Be Protective for Diabetes." *European Association for the Study of Diabetes 2014 Meeting* September 16, 2014; Vienna, Austria. Abstract 62.

Campbell, B.L., et al. "U.S. and Canadian Consumer Perception of Local and Organic Terminology." *International Food and Agribusiness Management Review* 17, no. 2 (2014).

Chowdhury, R., et al. "Association of Dietary, Circulating, and Supplement Fatty Acids with Coronary Risk: A Systematic Review and Meta-Analysis." *Annals of Internal Medicine* 160, no. 6 (18 Mar. 2014): pp. 398–406.

Deol, P., et al. "Soybean Oil Is More Obesogenic and Diabetogenic Than Coconut Oil and Fructose in Mouse: Potential Role for the Liver." *PLOS ONE* 10, no. 7 (22 Jul. 2015): p. e0132672.

Drake, I., et al. "Dietary Intakes of Carbohydrates in Relation to Prostate Cancer Risk: A Prospective Study in the Malmö Diet and Cancer Cohort." *American Journal of Clinical Nutrition* 96, no. 6 (2012): pp. 1409–18.

"Egg Consumption 'Positively Impacts Metabolic Syndrome and Satiety.'" *Yahoo News* (Apr. 2012).

Ferdman, R.A. "How Much Do Americans Love French Fries and Ketchup? A Lot More Than You Think." *The Washington Post* (21 Sep. 2015).

"Foods Identified as 'Whole Grain' Not Always Healthy." Harvard School of Public Health, http://www.hsph.harvard.edu/news/press-releases/foods-identified-as-whole-grain-not-always-healthy/.

Gibbons, L. "Food Prices 'Drive' Obesity Epidemic." *Foodmanufacture.co.uk.* Last updated May 11, 2015.

Gray, N. "Dietary Fat Plays Vital Role in Inflammatory Response and Obesity Related Disease Risk." *Foodnavigator.com.* Last updated September 28, 2015.

Herman, M.A. "The Role of ChREBP in Fructose Induced Metabolic Disease." Beth Israel Deaconess Medical Center. http://grantome.com/grant/NIH/R01-DK100425-01.

Hshieh, T.T., et al. "Nut Consumption and Risk of Mortality in the Physicians' Health Study." *American Journal of Clinical Nutrition* 101, no. 2 (2015): 407–412.

Jancin, B. "Low Carb Diet Didn't Boost CV Risk." *Skin and Allergy News Digital Network* (23 Jan. 2013).

Johnson, R.J. *The Sugar Fix.* New York: Simon and Schuster, 2008.

Jones, N.R.V., et al. "The Growing Price Gap between More and Less Healthy Foods: Analysis of a Novel Longitudinal UK Dataset." *PLOS ONE* (Oct. 2014).

Kothar, S.C., et al. "Subchronic Toxicity and Mutagenicity/Genotoxicity Studies of Irvingia Gabonensis Extract." *Food and Chemical Toxicology* 50, no. 5 (2012): pp. 1468–79.

Lawrence Kien, C., et al. "Lipidomic Evidence that Lowering the Typical Dietary Palmitate to Oleate Ratio in Humans Decreases the Leukocyte Production of Proinflammatory Cytokines and Muscle Expression of Redox-Sensitive Genes." *The Journal of Nutritional Biochemistry* 26, no. 12 (2015): pp. 1599–1606.

Muraki, I., et al. "Fruit Consumption and Risk of Type 2 Diabetes: Results From Three Prospective Longitudinal Cohort Studies." *BMJ* (29 Aug. 2013).

Ngondi, J.L., et al. "IGOB131, a Novel Seed Extract of the West African Plant Irvingia Gabonensis, Significantly Reduces Body Weight and Improves Metabolic Parameters in Overweight Humans in a Randomized Double-Blind Placebo Controlled Investigation." *Lipids in Health and Disease* 8 (2 Mar. 2009): p. 7. doi: 10.1186/1476-511X-8-7.

Ngondi, J.L., et al. "The Effect of Irvingia Gabonensis Seeds on Body Weight and Blood Lipids of Obese Subjects in Cameroon." *Lipids in Health and Disease* (2005). https://www.ncbi.nlm.nih.gov/pmc/articles/PMC1168905/.

Pan, A., et al. "Walnut Consumption Is Associated with Lower Risk of Type 2 Diabetes in Women." *Journal of Nutrition* 143, no. 4 (Apr. 2013): pp. 512–18.

Prescott, B. "New Research Could Pave the Way for Fructose Tolerance Test." *Beth Israel Deaconess Medical Center* (2014). http://www.bidmc.org/News/In-Research/2014/October/Fructose.aspx.

Pu, S., et al. "Interactions Between Dietary Oil Treatments and Genetic Variants Modulate Fatty Acid Ethanolamides in Plasma and Body Weight Composition." *British Journal of Nutrition* 115, no. 6 (Mar. 2016).

Roberts, R.O., et al. "Relative Intake of Macronutrients Impacts Risk of Mild Cognitive Impairment or Dementia." *Journal of Alzheimers Disease* 32, no. 2 (2012): pp. 329–39.

Robinson, N. "Drug Link Would Increase Fruit and Veg Consumption." *Food Manufacture* (1 Oct. 2014).

Ruff, J.S., et al. "Compared to Sucrose, Previous Consumption of Fructose and Glucose Monosaccharides Reduces Survival and Fitness of Female Mice." *Journal of Nutrition* 145, no. 3 (2015): pp. 434–41.

Sack, D. "4 Ways Sugar Could be Harming Your Mental Health." *Psychology Today* (2013). Posted September 2, 2013. https://www.psychologytoday.com/blog/where-science-meets-the-steps/201309/4-ways-sugar-could-be-harming-your-mental-health.

"Sugar and 'Bad' Carbs Cause Early Signs of Dementia." *Natural Health Advisory* (Oct. 2012).

Taubes, G. "What If It's All Been a Big Fat Lie?" *New York Times* (7 Jun. 2002).

Tucker, M.E. "Tree Nuts Improve Glycemic Control in Type 2 Diabetes." *PLOS ONE* (30 Jul. 2014).

Viguiliouk, E., et al. "Effect of Tree Nuts on Glycemic Control in Diabetes: A Systematic Review and Meta-Analysis of Randomized Controlled Dietary Trials." *PLOS ONE* 9, no. 7 (2014).

Wang, X., et al. "Fruit and Vegetable Consumption and Mortality From All Causes, Cardiovascular Disease, and Cancer: Systematic Review and Dose-Response Meta-Analysis of Prospective Cohort Studies." *BMJ* (29 Jul. 2014).

Wiggins, S., et al. "The Rising Cost of a Healthy Diet: Changing Relative Prices of Foods in High-Income and Emerging Economies." Odi.org (May 2015).

Yang, Q., et al. "Added Sugar Intake and Cardiovascular Diseases Mortality Among US Adults." *JAMA* 174, no. 4 (Apr. 2014): pp. 516–24.

CHAPTER 8

Alzheimer's Association International Conference (*AAIC*) 2014. Presented 14 Jul. 2014.

Buijsse, Brian, et al. "Physical Activity and Mortality in Individuals With Diabetes Mellitus: A Prospective Study and Meta-analysis." *JAMA, Archives of Internal Medicine* (6 Aug. 2012): pp. 1–11.

Cassels, C. "Any Level of Midlife Exercise May Keep Dementia at Bay." Medscape (17 Jul. 2014).

Cherkas L.F., et al. "The Association Between Physical Activity in Leisure Time and Leukocyte Telomere Length." *JAMA, Archives of Internal Medicine* 168, no. 2 (2008): pp. 154–58.

Freeman, D.W. "Too Much Sitting behind 92,000 Cancer Cases a Year: Report." *CBS News* (3 Nov. 2011). Accessed 14 Jan. 2014.

Grøntved, A., et al. "A Prospective Study of Weight Training and Risk of Type 2 Diabetes Mellitus in Men" *JAMA, Archives of Internal Medicine* (6 Aug. 2012): pp. 1–7.

Henson, J., et al. "Associations of Objectively Measured Sedentary Behaviour and Physical Activity With Markers of Cardiometabolic Health." *Diabetologia* 56, no. 5 (May 2013): pp. 1012–20.

Internicola, D. "Trying to Lose Weight? Ditch Calorie-Rich Rewards after Exercise." *Reuters* (22 Jul. 2013).

Katz, M.H. "Writing More Specific Exercise Prescriptions." *JAMA, Archives of Internal Medicine* (6 Aug. 2012): pp. 1–2.

Katzmarzyk, P.T., et al. "Sedentary Behaviour and Life Expectancy in the USA: A Cause-Deleted Life Table Analysis." *BMJ Open* 2, no. 4 (2012).

LaRocca, T.J., et al. "Leukocyte Telomere Length is Preserved with Aging in Endurance Exercise-Trained Adults and Related to Maximal Aerobic

Capacity." *Mechanisms of Ageing and Development* 131, no. 2 (Feb. 2010): pp. 165–7.

Laverty, A.A., et al. "Active Travel to Work and Cardiovascular Risk Factors in the United Kingdom." *American Journal of Preventive Medicine* 45, no. 3 (Sep. 2013): pp. 282–88.

Mansikkamäki, K., et al. "Physical Activity and Menopause-Related Quality of Life: A Population-Based Cross-Sectional Study." *Maturitas* 80, no. 1 (2015): pp. 69–74.

Mavros, Y., et al. "Changes in Insulin Resistance and HbA1c Are Related to Exercise-Mediated Changes in Body Composition in Older Adults with Type 2 Diabetes: Interim Outcomes from the GREAT2DO Trial." *Diabetes Care* (8 Mar. 2013).

Nelson, Jennifer K. "Do You Have 'Sitting Disease?'" *Mayo Clinic* (25 Jun. 2012). Accessed 17 Jan. 2014.

Puterman, E., et al. "The Power of Exercise: Buffering the Effect of Chronic Stress on Telomere Length." *PLOS ONE* 5, no. 5 (26 May 2010).

Reynolds, G. "How Exercising Keeps Your Cells Young." *New York Times* (27 Jan. 2010).

Seguin, R., et al. "Sedentary Behavior and Mortality in Older Women." *American Journal of Preventive Medicine* (Jan. 2014).

Simon, R.M., et al. "The Association of Exercise with Both Erectile and Sexual Function in Black and White Men." *Journal of Sexual Medicine* (20 Mar. 2015).

Stensvold, D., et al. "Effect of Exercise Training on Inflammation Status Among People With Metabolic Syndrome." *Metabolic Syndrome and Related Disorders* 10, no. 4 (2012): pp. 267–72.

Werner, C., et al. "Abstract 1380: Beneficial Effects of Long-Term Endurance Exercise on Leukocyte Telomere Biology." *Circulation* (3 Nov. 2009).

Yates, T., et al. "Association between Change in Daily Ambulatory Activity and Cardiovascular Events in People with Impaired Glucose Tolerance (NAVIGATOR Trial): A Cohort Analysis." *Lancet* 383, no. 9922 (19 Dec. 2013).

CHAPTER 10

Burger, K.S., et al. "Frequent Ice Cream Consumption Is Associated with Reduced Striatal Response to Receipt of an Ice Cream-Based Milkshake." *The American Journal of Clinical Nutrition* 95, no. 4 (Apr. 2012): pp. 810–17.

Cohen M.R., et al. "Naloxone Reduces Food Intake in Humans." *Psychosom Medicine* 47, no. 2 (Mar.–Apr. 1985): pp. 132–38.

Connecticut College. "Are Oreos Addictive? Research Says Yes." *ScienceDaily* (15 Oct. 2013).

"Effects of Dietary Glycemic Index on Brain Regions Related to Reward and Craving in Men." *American Journal of Clinical Nutrition* (26 Jun. 2013): doi: 10.3945/ajcn.113.064113

"Effects of Fructose vs. Glucose on Regional Cerebral Blood Flow in Brain Regions Involved with Appetite and Reward Pathways." *JAMA* 309, no. 1 (2013): pp. 63–70.

Recipe Index

General Index

About the Author

FRED PESCATORE, MD, is a traditionally trained physician practicing nutritional medicine in Manhattan. He is the author of several books, including the *New York Times* best-seller *The Hamptons Diet* and the number-one best-selling children's health book *Feed Your Kids Well*.

Prior to opening his own practice, Dr. Pescatore worked closely with the late, great Dr. Robert C. Atkins, as the Associate Medical Director of the Atkins Center for Complementary Medicine.

"Dr. Fred" is internationally recognized as a health, nutrition, and weight loss expert. He is president of the International and American Association of Clinical Nutritionists and a member of the American College for the Advancement of Medicine, and belongs to many other professional organizations.

He is a regular contributor to *In Touch, Us Weekly, First for Women*, and *Women's World* magazines. Major network television shows like *Extra, The View, Rachael Ray*, and *Today* have sought out Dr. Pescatore for his expert health advice. His practice has become a haven for the rich and famous, drawing a roster of clientele that reads like a "Who's Who" of Hollywood's elite.

Dr. Pescatore is also deeply involved in the philanthropic community, devoting time to working in hospitals in developing nations around the world, as well as helping support various health organizations across this country.

Join the A-List for FREE at AListDietBook.com

Dear Reader,

Want the latest A-List tips and tricks that are working *right now* for my celebrity clients?

Go to AListDietBook.com and get all this for FREE:

- ✓ **The A-List Celebrity Cheat Sheet for Even Faster Results**
- ✓ **Personalized A-List advice—tailored just for you and your weight loss goals**
- ✓ **Bonus quizzes to help you find out which type of "A-Lister" you are**
- ✓ **Exclusive discounts on new products designed to make The A-List Diet even easier!**

You'll find these insider perks (and more!) only at AListDietBook.com.

See you there!

—DR. FRED